Living While Dying

Benita C. Martocchio, Ph.D., R.N.

**Associate Professor, Medical/Surgical Nursing,
Case Western Reserve University, Cleveland, Ohio
Clinical Associate, University Hospitals of Cleveland**

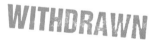

Robert J. Brady Co., Bowie, Md.
A Prentice-Hall Publishing and Communications Co.

Executive Producer: Richard A. Weimer
Production Editor: Paula K. Aldrich
Art Director: Don Sellers

Living while dying.

Library of Congress Cataloging in Publication Data

Martocchio, Benita C., 1934-
    Living while dying.

    Includes bibliographical references and index.
        1. Terminal care.   2. Terminally ill.
I. Title.   [DNLM: 1. Attitude to death.
BF 789.D4 M387s]
R726.8.M37   362.1'7   81-6081
ISBN 0-87619-922-8   AACR2

Prentice-Hall International, Inc., London
Prentice-Hall of Australia, Pty., Ltd., Sydney
Prentice-Hall of India Private Limited, New Delhi
Prentice-Hall of Japan, Inc., Tokyo
Prentice-Hall of Southeast Asia Pte. Ltd., Singapore
Whitehall Books, Limited, Petone, New Zealand

Printed in the United States of America

82 83 84 85 86 87 88 89 90 91 92   10 9 8 7 6 5 4 3 2

CONTENTS

FOREWORD

Dr. Martocchio's study of dying patients is concerned with human behavior in interaction with the environment during the critical life situation of dying. The focus of the book is on the social and psychological processes at work among people who are *living* while dying and those persons interacting with them. It is a book that will be of great value not only to nurses, sociologists, social workers, and health professionals at all levels, but to all people concerned with the dying experience. Her book provides us with substantive help both in the delivery of health care to individuals, and in understanding the sociological implications of this unique life experience. Her study demonstrates ways to foster self-caring behavior that leads to individual health and well being during the dying process.

Her book comes at a crucial time for nursing because of the need to identify the uniqueness of nursing science and practice in today's health care system, especially in the rapidly expanding hospice movement. Her study identifies a structured body of knowledge for nurses and others to use in assisting a dying individual within his or her environment. The close relationship between knowledge gained for the academic discipline of nursing and this knowledge serving as a basis for professional practice is evident. This book should aid in the public's and the profession's understanding of the social relevance of nursing. I could not help but rejoice at the legitimacy of nursing that comes through so clearly for society and the imperative demand for nursing to demonstrate leadership skills in the care of the dying patient and family.

Her first chapter, on dying and death in past generations, is by far the best I have read among the explosion of books in this area. It was refreshing to read and learn new information; her synthesis of the vast amount of material is excellent and gives a rich appreciation of the generations past in Western thought and cultures. Her coverage of how death became a social problem in the twentieth century is very well done for she grapples with the many dilemmas present, and presents a most logical and meaningful chapter.

I quote: "If people gained competence in dealing with terminating relationships throughout their lives, they should be better able to maintain interactional relationships preceding death. If there is to be a quality of living during this living-while-knowingly-dying period, the continuation or discontinuation of interactional relationships should be based upon mutual decision. It should not be due to a lack of competence in interacting in the situation nor to poorly defined role expectations." Her book should aid all of us to gain competence.

I was delighted to read that her data collection took two years. Data collection should take time. I am deeply concerned over doctoral students who get all their data collected in two months. The complexity of research requires considerable time and also taking advantage of the multiple data sources available.

Chapter 5 includes the description of the patient, staff, and disease conditions. Included here are patterns of living-dying with pictorial representations of variations, which is a more accurate portrayal of the dying trajectories than developed by earlier researchers. Chapter 6 makes clear the distinction between those with a high risk of dying and those who are actually dying. The figure of transitional states provides a helpful model for teaching students and practitioners the relationships in which one works daily. This chapter provides rich data that document the crucial involvement of nursing; her choice of examples is clear and convincing. Chapter 7 should be used by physicians to realize the inappropriateness of some of their demands and role expectations during the dying phase. The physician cannot be all things to the patient and the family—how much more appropriate it is for the care providers to give the needed support to the family and the dying patient. Certainly the physician needs to support nurses, just as nurses need to support physicians so that all effectively work together for the sake of public health needs.

The last chapter on the realities of dying sums up much of what dying patients and families tell us. Her description of detached concern includes aspects that will make the term more concrete for care providers. A term I have personally used is "detached compassion" to explain the same requirement of the care providers. An additional term that could be used in this closing chapter is "comfort care," a term meant to describe the changes in care requirement as the patient nears the end of life and the comfort care requirements supersede those of cure-oriented care. Her book adds much to the concept of comfort care in the interaction of persons in both the psychological and sociological aspects. This needs to be meshed with the physiological needs of the patient and a more total care will result.

This is a book that will aid all those concerned with the dying experience, whether they are the immediate interactors in a health care situation or the active researchers engaged in studying this human phenomenon. It will provide a better framework for understanding the various situations encountered in living-while-dying, and also prove to be a stimulus for further research and inquiry into this little known but profoundly interesting area of human experience.

Hong Kong, Sept. 1980

Ida M. Martinson Ph.D., F.A.A.N.
Professor & Director of Research
School of Nursing
University of Minnesota

PREFACE

Dying and death are here to stay. They will not vanish. Despite the amazing advances of science, medical knowledge, and technology, dying is and will remain an integral part of living.

This is a report of a study about people dying in hospitals. The focus is upon the social and psychological processes and factors that impinge upon people living their dying and those interacting with them.

This book will be of interest to all who have wondered about dying, their own or that of others. It is based upon the experiences of 47 people living their dying, and of their families, friends, and health care providers. It was written to acquaint readers with some of the wide ranges of experiences and factors associated with living while dying.

Each chapter focuses upon a different aspect of living with dying. Although each chapter fully addresses a selected topic and readers are free to select according to their interests, they should keep in mind that each chapter speaks to only a part of the total situation.

People have always had to cope with the eventuality of death. Chapter 1 focuses on the changing beliefs and attitudes people have held toward dying and death from primitive times until the present. Throughout history, people have manifested a persistent desire to believe that death is not the absolute end and that life after death is not an illusion; but never in history have dying and death created greater problems than in the twentieth century. Chapter 2 focuses upon the twentieth century by addressing death as a social problem. This chapter includes prevailing attitudes and behaviors associated with dying and death. It touches on some of the larger issues associated with dying, e.g., living wills, definitions of death, quality of life. The second half of the chapter consists of studies of persons facing imminent death.

Chapter 3 focuses on several theoretical and sensitizing concepts drawn from the literature and also upon the objectives and questions guiding this research. Chapter 4 tells how this research was done. A description of the hospital and all the interactors is presented in Chapter 5. Major emphasis is on describing the patients, their characteristics and their patterns of living-dying.

Chapters 6 and 7 address the major research questions. Conversations are presented, analyzed, and explained. These conversations can be used as data for study or guides to care.

Chapter 8 serves as a unifying chapter. It addresses the realities of dying from the perspectives of those living their dying, of their family members, and of their health care providers.

The completion of this study is attributable to the efforts of many people who have given generously of their time, ideas, and concern. As a sociologist, practicing nurse clinician, and faculty member of the School of Nursing, Case Western Reserve University, I have been fortunate to have access to many health care facilities and have been able to observe, interview, and exchange ideas with many health care providers, researchers, faculty members, and students. Although it is not possible to name each person, I am grateful to all of them, as well as to my former professors, especially Irwin Deutscher, Sharon Guten, Marie Haug, Lloyd Rogler, and Marvin B. Sussman.

I express my appreciation to my family and friends who helped in innumerable ways to make this book a reality. I am especially indebted to Charlene Phelps, whose research commitment made data collection for this study possible; and to Wilma J. Phipps for sharing her expertise and investing many hours in editing the final copy. I also thank Virginia Cassmeyer, Barbara Daly, James Dickoff, Karin Dufault, S.P., Rosemary Ellis, Patricia James, Jannetta MacPhail, Antoinette Ragucci, and Betty Rautio for their contributions, suggestions, stimulating comments, and questions; and Rev. Paul Martinson, Rozella Scholtfeldt, and Charles Schmitz, S.J., for their suggestions about Chapter One. Thanks are also extended to Jeannette Kaufman and Sondra Patrizzi for typing and retyping the manuscript.

Most of all, I thank the patients, their families, and the health care providers who participated in this research.

Benita C. Martocchio

With Love and Respect
To My Parents,
Ben and Mildred Martocchio

1   Dying and Death in Past Generations

Dying and death are two associated concepts. They are so closely associated that it is difficult to think about dying without thinking about death. There are some important differences, however. Dying refers to the *process* of nearing or coming to an end and is an integral part of living, while death is an *event*—the end of physical life—the permanent cessation of all vital functions.

Although admittedly an empirical question, it is possible that if many people view death as an abnormal and abhorrent event, so may they also view dying. What then happens to dying persons? Are they viewed as abhorrent persons who should be isolated from others? Do dying people experience a type of social death long before they experience physical death? Must dying be seen as a terrible process? What factors contribute to peoples' perceptions of dying and thus their behaviors when faced with dying?

History is one factor that contributes to behavior. Although there is debate about whether everyone can accept dying as an integral part of living, there is a relationship between the way people live and the way people die. In describing the interrelationships between major cultural patterns of living and funeral practices, Ruth Benedict (1) notes that the way an individual faces dying and deals with death represents the prevailing values of the society or group of people to which the individual belongs. These prevailing values or beliefs shape both how each individual views dying and death and how each individual copes with them.

The values or beliefs of any society or any individual are embedded in history. Thus, knowing the history of attitudes, beliefs, and practices related to dying and death contributes to understanding the basis for some of the fears, dilemmas, and practices associated with dying and death in contemporary society. More importantly, a historical perspective contributes to better understanding what the people in the study were experiencing and trying to communicate. The influence of history is reflected in their religious beliefs, attitudes and expectations, use of folklore, and behavioral practices.

History offers some possible solutions to the problems and dilemmas associated with dying. For example, hospice is a medieval concept which is being explored as one way to care for the dying. Thus, understanding of what has gone before may assist in identifying ways to better cope with dying and care for the dying. In addition, a brief review of history contributes to understanding both the similarities and the differences between past and contemporary views and practices, as well as to understanding the contrasts and conflicts which prevail in contemporary society.

Although fear of dying and death is generally recognized as a universal phenomenon (2), authors (3) suggest that members of contemporary industrialized societies experience greater anxiety and anguish related to dying and death than people of earlier times. Dying and death are matters relegated to books, articles, or special television programs, but are considered in poor taste as topics for discussion in every day conversation. In fact, in contemporary industrialized societies a number of authors (4) have described the very topics of dying and death as taboo.

Dying and death were not always seen as "taboo" subjects, nor were they always considered problems needing study. Yet, people have always had to cope with the eventuality of death. All cultures, even the most primitive ones, have evolved beliefs concerning death, its cause and significance. Over time, there has been a slow and almost imperceptible change in beliefs and accompanying attitudes. People continue to be concerned about the nature of death and the purpose of life. Although they continue to manifest a persistent desire to believe that death is not the absolute end and that life after death is not an illusion, views and behaviors differ.

PRIMITIVE SOCIETIES

In the earliest stages of human development, death was seen as accidental, not inevitable. Primitive people believed that humans were created immortal. When death occurred, it was attributed to something other than natural causes and was not seen as the end of life. Primitive people made no connection between aging, loss of bodily functioning or general progressive debilitation, and dying. Death occurred as a result of an accident, was self-inflicted, or caused by an enemy in either human or spiritual form. Sickness was attributed to magical powers or to the intervention of a mystical force (5). In other words, primitive people believed that if it were not for accidents or magically induced illnesses, no one would ever die (6). Myths of primitive people about the origin of death reflect these beliefs (7).

The causes and significance of death were not of major concern. Since primitive people believed they knew the cause of death, there was no reason to search fot it (8). When death did occur, it was viewed as a crisis to be endured before entering a new status (9). Death was something that happened *to* them. It was viewed as an event, just as birth, growing up, and marriage are events in life. The idea that death was inevitable, or that people themselves might be responsible for their own deaths, was not found among primitives (10). Curious as it may seem, primitive people did not view death as inevitable, even though they witnessed it frequently.

There is controversy over how people discovered that death is inevitable. Choron (11) suggests that there are two necessary conditions leading to the discovery of the inevitability of death. The first condition is the process of individualization. In individualization there is a change from the primitive view of seeing oneself as being part of a clan or a horde with the most important characteristic being one's place in the group, to an awareness of oneself as an individual with characteristics of his own. The second condition is the ability to reason logically. In Choron's view, once the conditions of individualization and logical reasoning are met, the individual could conclude that all people are mortal and realize that he, too, has to die.

Although Choron's explanation has been challenged by others, the important factor is that people did realize that death was inevitable and this discovery brought its own fears and anxieties. However, primitive people were still protected from the fear of total annihilation by their unquestioned beliefs that death was not absolute and that immortality was a certainty (12). No one died completely. People changed from one form to another and communicated in different ways but they continued to live while waiting for reincarnation.

These beliefs persist among members of contemporary primitive societies. For example, the notion of the lack of finality of death is seen in the Tasmanian and Samoan belief that people possess a soul that lives after death in the form of a ghost which retains all the characteristics of the living person. These ghosts are in essence each person's spiritual double (13).

Experts who examined mythology in depth describe the certainty of the belief in immortality: ". . . death is universally found to be part of a cycle of death and rebirth, or to be the condition necessary to imagine transcendence of life in an experience of resurrection (14)." Their findings support those of Murdock (15) who described the polar Eskimos' belief that people have two spiritual attributes, a name and a soul. After death the name leaves the corpse and enters the body of a pregnant woman and is reborn in the child. Ducasse (16) describes a variation of the belief among the tribesmen of central Australia who believe that after death the spirit of the dead person remains near its former home, waiting for the opportunity to enter a pregnant woman so that it can be reborn. The reborn tribesmen then live a life similar to their former existence. Pregnant women, somewhat ambivalent about this belief, shy away from places where such spirits might be found.

It is impossible to determine precisely when people abandoned belief in the imperishability of the human personality. It is more a story of growing skepticism and a gradual abandonment of the belief by a majority of the members of society. Actually, the primitive conceptions of life after death, in particular the birth, death, and rebirth notions, continue to exist alongside Jewish and Christian traditions of contemporary Western societies.

Reincarnation is presently a subject of great interest to some and scholars are seriously studying it (17). Using spirits or ghosts as characters of fiction is an accepted practice (18), as is the reincarnation of major characters (19). Burying toys or prized possessions with the dead remains popular among some members of industrialized societies (20). These practices show a persistent belief in the permanence or indestructibility of the human personality, even though there has been a gradual abandonment of this view by members of contemporary society. Just as some of the beliefs and characteristics of primitive cultures persist today, other elements of current thought have arisen from beliefs held by ancient societies, such as that of the Egyptians.

ANTIQUITY

The ancient Eygptians developed a complex intellectual and technological society. The basic conditions of their lives, however, were not different from those that prevailed throughout early history. Life expectancy was short and people rarely lived beyond early maturity. Deaths among infants and children were expected, as were deaths from childbirth. Few persons survived into advanced years, and thus few deaths were attributed to old age. In fact, persons of advanced age, who retained their mental and physical prowess wielded considerable social influence (21).

Generally, the Egyptians' hold on life was precarious. They had little control over the forces of nature and, as a result, life was mysterious and unpredictable. As evidenced in their myths and practices, ancient people wished to control their environment but, unlike today, they did not expect to be able to do so.

Dying and death were visible. People witnessed death often. Since continuity of life was achieved through the extended family or the clan or tribe, the fate of the individual was not of primary importance. Individuals were important only in terms of their performance within and their obligations to the group. The person was primarily a social component who performed according to the dictates of custom.

The Egyptian Book of the Dead (22), written in 1600 B.C., provided a detailed account of burial practices. It offered a guide for dealing with death during a time which might have promoted a feeling of helplessness. It treated the journey of the human soul into eternity as a certainty. The Egyptian belief in the certainty of an afterlife may be interpreted in several ways. It may represent a means of assuring people some control over their situation; it may represent a defense against viewing death as total annihilation; or it may be an expression of the belief of human indestructibility.

About 1200 B.C., views toward death changed and skepticism replaced certainty. A strong element of doubt about the existence of a future life was in evidence and a new conception arose concerning what might happen to the person after death (23). Future life, if it existed, was not seen as being in touch with or related to the past life, but was seen as "a·release from this life and a reward for humble patience in this life (24)." Life after death was earned; it was no longer a certainty for all. Thus, death was absolute and inevitable and man was mortal.

With the recognition of the possibility that death was not only inevitable but absolute, dying and death became matters of deep concern. Life after death became a hope, not an unquestioned certainty. Fear of dying and the sense of futility of life became intense. Although the ancient Greeks stressed the joys of life, they were very much aware of the uncertainties and the transitory nature of life and of the imminence of death (25). The ancient Greeks saw the world as beautiful and, in contrast, they saw death as a terrible and frightening end of the human condition. Death was accepted with melancholy resignation.

Antiquity marked the beginning of an acute consciousness of human mortality—a consciousness which persisted throughout the ages and is no less acute in contemporary industrial societies. The Greeks exemplified ancient people's struggle with their desire to believe that death was not the absolute end and that life after death was not an illusion. During antiquity skepticism towards the assertion of myths and prevailing religious doctrine grew. Death was a cause for concern, a problem with two main aspects—the mastery of fear of death and the meaning of human existence. During this period, death generally was regarded as a fearsome and evil thing, a great misfortune which aroused a variety of emotions and attitudes (26). Although fearsome, it was seen as an inevitable and inescapable part of life. The emergence of a different view of immortality, the immortality of the soul, offered some consolation. This view offered a reasonable and plausible hope for immortality, not a certainty as believed during previous ages.* Solace was gained from the belief that death opened the door to a new and better life.

DEATH AND THE BIBLE

No overview of the historical perspective of dying and death would be complete without some discussion of the conception of death as presented in the Bible. Over the centuries, views of death have been influenced by changing theological doctrines. The Christian view of death has held a monopoly for nearly two thousand years in Western civilizations and continues to find wide acceptance. Scientists and philosophers who have been reluctant to accept Christian beliefs are known to take refuge in them when death is close at hand (27).

THE OLD TESTAMENT

The early Hebrews, like other ancients, believed in magical powers and in the existence of supernatural beings. They differed from their ancient counterparts in two important ways. First, they believed in one God who was the source of all life; and second, they believed that misfortune, such as disease, disaster, and death, resulted from disobeying God (28). They believed that misdeeds of a community could bring plague and pestilence upon an entire nation.

The Hebrews viewed death as an inevitable fact of life. As a consequence, they were resigned to their fate. The following quotations taken from the Old Testament illustrate this view.

> The Lord from earth created man,
>   and in his image made him.
> Limited days of life he gives him
>   and makes him return to earth again (29).

> All flesh grown old, like a garment:
>   the age old law is: all must die.
> As with the leaves that grow on a
>   vigorous tree: one falls off and another sprouts—
> So with generations of flesh, and blood:
>   one died and another is born (30).

> We must indeed die; we are then like water that is poured out on the ground and cannot be gathered up. Yet, though God does not bring back life, he does take thought how not to banish anyone from him (31).

The Old Testament offers little consolation for the fact of death in terms of life after death. Most of the books of the Old Testament do not present a concept of a true life after death. Ecclesiastes is probably representative.

> Go thy way, eat thy bread with joy, and drink thy wine with a merry heart; for God now accepteth thy works. Whatsoever thy hand findeth to do,

---

*For a detailed account of Plato's arguments, especially in Phaedo, see Taylor AE, *Plato, the Man and His Work*, New York, Meridian Books, 1956, pp. 183 – 207.

do it with thy might; for there is no work, nor devise, no knowledge, nor wisdom, in the grave, whither thou goest. (32).

If little solace is to be found in a belief in life after death, there is less to be found in the Old Testament's account of the origin of death. According to the Old Testament, "God saw everything that He made and He found it very good (33)." He created people to live and not to die. People brought anything evil, including death, upon themselves; God was blameless (34). As a consequence, a sense of guilt was inherent and fears of retribution reinforced.

The notion that the Lord will postpone death for the repentant sinner so that he may fulfill his destiny of praising God on earth offered some comfort (35). Understanding death at a young age became a more perplexing problem than death itself.

Once I said,
"In the noontime of life I must depart
To the gates of neither world I shall be consigned
for the rest of my years (36)."

. . . I say: O my God
Take me not hence in the midst of my days;
through all generations your years endure (37).

One possible solution to the problem of God's willing premature death was sought in making it a consequence of sin.

For each man's ways are plain to the Lord's sight;
all their paths he surveys;
By his own iniquities the wicked man will be caught,
in the meshes of his own sin he will be held fast.
He will die from lack of discipline,
through the greatness of his folly he will be lost (38).

And you, O God, will bring them down
into the pit of destruction;
Men of blood and deceit shall not live
out half their lives (39).

Reflect now, what innocent person perishes?
Since when are the upright destroyed?
As I see it, those who plow for mischief and
sow trouble, reap the same.
By the breath of God they perish, and by the
blast of his wrath they are consumed (40).

Nevertheless, the recognition that the young died while the wicked survived, grew old, and became mighty in power (41), evoked anguish and uncertainty.

Where was solace to be found among the authors of the Old Testament? There is little mention of life beyond death. The authors offered at best a kind of continuity through one's children. Death was presented as the heaviest burden of human existence, a penalty for sin brought upon man by man. Comfort was found in faith, trust, and reliance upon an all-powerful creator expressed in an unquestioned acceptance of God's will: ". . . The Lord giveth, and the Lord taketh away: blessed be the name of the Lord (42)." Comfort also was found in the growing conviction that all things are possible for God (43): ". . . he will destroy death forever. The Lord God will wipe away the tears from all faces (44)."

It would be erroneous to conclude that the idea of life after death and resurrection are completely absent in the Old Testament. Although the greater part of the Old Testament looked upon death as a curse, it yearned for a life after death that embraced the *whole person*, not an immortality of *the soul* as espoused by the Greeks. The following passages hint at this tendency toward a concept of resurrection.

Isaiah stated:

But your dead shall live, their corpses shall rise;
    awake and sing, you who lie in the dust.
For your dew is a dew of light,
    and the land of shades gives birth (45).

Daniel wrote:

Many of those who sleep
    in the dust of the earth shall awake;
Some shall live forever,
    Others shall be an ever lasting horror and
    disgrace (46).

Even Job offered some hope:

But as for me, I know that my Vindicator lives,
    and that he will at last stand forth upon the dust
Whom I myself shall see:
    my own eyes, not another's shall behold him.
And from my flesh I shall see God;
    my inmost being is consumed with longing (47).

The ancient Greeks pondered the meaning of human life as related to death. Similarly, the whole Book of Job, written in approximately 400 B.C., explores the meaning of suffering by raising timely questions. Is individual suffering always the direct result of sinfulness? Should suffering be questioned or should it be used constructively as an atonement for one's own or the sins of others? Instead of answers, Job offers assurance that there is a God who will help people to rise above suffering and pain and that even in the face of suffering and pain, there is meaning to living a righteous life.

The Book of Wisdom, which was composed and edited in Greek by a Jewish scholar in Alexandria, Egypt, one or two hundred years before the coming of Christ, added another dimension to the thoughts about suffering, death and life after death. The author redefined the meaning of suffering and offered an "escape" from spiritual death. Although alluded to in other parts of the Old Testament, the Book of Wisdom contains the earliest explicit statement about life after death, and the word "immortality" appears for the first time in scripture (48).

Although death was still viewed by some as a punishment for sin and wrongdoing and long life the reward of virtue, it was possible to escape from death, at least from spiritual death. Through virtue people could achieve immortality (49). The notion that suffering was an indication of God's punishment for evildoing was dismissed. Instead, the Book of Wisdom teaches that although the righteous may appear to be punished in the "sight of man," there is a beneficial purpose to their suffering in the "sight of God." "Chastised a little, they shall be greatly blessed, because God tried them and found them worthy of himself (50)." Perhaps of major importance in resolving the dilemma associated with premature death was the teaching that people must not measure their lives by length but rather by the quality of life lived in the time given them (51).

> You have been told, O man, what is good,
> and what the Lord requires of you:
> Only to do right and to love goodness,
> and to walk humbly with your God (52).

THE NEW TESTAMENT

The New Testament is the story of the conquering of death through the paradox of a better life coming through death. It offered the bold promise of resurrection of the body as well as the spirit (53). It was the answer to the persistent desire to believe that death was not the absolute end and that life after death was not an illusion.

The spreading of the "Good News" of salvation began during a period when there was great preoccupation with death and the fear of death (54). People actively sought escape from and solutions to the problems of death by focusing on the meaning of life and the assurance of immortality. The Hebrews found comfort in their complete reliance upon the will of God. The Pharisees held firmly to their belief in the resurrection of the dead. Philosophers were preoccupied with debates about immortality, the Romans relied upon rituals for assuring life everlasting. The concern of the Romans was so great that mysterious rites for preparing the body were usual and the sale of pills alleged to assure life after death became a lucrative business (55). The world was ready for this proclamation of victory over death which was anticipated in the Old Testament (56) and which was promised in the teachings of Jesus of Nazareth (57).

Although history is marked by various doctrines of life after death none offered so complete and joyful a belief as that presented in the New Testament. As in the Old Testament, the origin of death was attributed to the sins of man, in particular to the first man, Adam (58). Similarly, the dead are withdrawn from any relation to God; however, by rising from the dead, Christ conquered death. Paul stated: "We know that Christ, once raised from the dead, will never die again; death has no more power over him (59)." Although human death was accepted as inevitable, it was also accepted as a certainty that "in Christ all will come to life again (60)." The option for a life everlasting was open to all who believed and who were willing to receive the Spirit through baptism (61).

The New Testament granted an even greater promise as at the end of time the victory over death would be complete. The dead will rise glorious and immortal (62). Although immortality of the soul was a familiar concept to the Greeks, the resurrection of the body was foreign to their thinking. When Paul was preaching in Athens he was sneered at when he mentioned the rising of the dead (63).

8

What occurred during this period between physical death and the victory over death? Paul's letter to the Thessalonians (64) explained this period as a kind of falling asleep in Christ, a state from which one would rise and meet the Lord.

The New Testament is the story of God's love for his people (65). It is the story of death as the consummation of the love of Christ (66). By dying on the cross, Jesus achieved the expiation for sin which was sought after but left unachieved in the Old Testament (67). It is the promise of the salvation of the world through the death and resurrection of Christ.

For the devout Christian no further explanation or proof was required beyond the views presented in the New Testament. Christ has died, Christ is risen, therefore people shall rise in Christ; thus, through death comes eternal life. There was no need to fear annihilation of the person and once again a future life was a certainty. When these beliefs prevailed, death was seen as a crisis. It was a temporary crisis, however, a necessary and preparatory event for another more glorious life. "Be glad and rejoice," says Matthew, "for your reward is great in heaven (68)."

The Early Christians. Over the centuries there has been considerable variation on the Christian view of death. It is possible to distinguish an early Christian view from a view characteristic of the Middle Ages (69).

The early Christians were not so concerned with the death of an individual as they were concerned about the end of the world which they saw as imminent. They focused attention upon Christ's promise that He would come again and call His elect from the ends of the earth. This Second Coming was perceived as a triumphal event, the vindication of those loyal followers who remained true to Him. As such, it was a source of hope, joy, and consolation. Of particular value to this small and persecuted group was their strong sense of community. They viewed the fate of the individual as inextricably bound to the fate of the community. They believed that theirs was a "saved" community destined for salvation. Their belief in salvation as a community was consistent with their life-style since during those days of persecution, only those who were faithful remained in the Christian community.

These early Christians found no terror in death. They looked forward to a new and better life after death: a resurrection of the body and a life of glory in eternal worship of God.

The Gospels also provided the basis for a different view of death including damnation—the shadowy life of the underworld or the life of a disembodied spirit. There are strong and repeated warnings that the Son of Man will come when least expected and for those who are taken unawares and unprepared, the coming of Christ would be a tragedy, not a triumph (70).

The minds of the early Christians were not encumbered by fears of eternal torture generated by these warnings. Harassed by persecution and in constant danger, they were not likely to forget to watch and pray.

THE MIDDLE AGES

THE EARLY MIDDLE AGES

The Christian view toward death gradually changed. Although the belief of a common destiny held by early Christians prevailed during the early Middle Ages, there was growing concern for the destiny of the individual. This increasing concern was reflected in the patterns of behavior surrounding dying. The pious prepared for death with ceremony. The ritual was basically religious, well known and followed by everyone probably because it was familiar and also because people held similar views of death.

Traditionally, the ceremony began with the Christian assuming the posture for dying: lying supine so that his or her face was turned toward heaven. The dying person lamented dying, reflected about loved ones and things, pardoned and perhaps asked pardon from friends, associates, family members, and the helpers who surrounded the deathbed, and commended them to God. There was the "culpa" or confession followed by the granting of absolution by the priest. The priest prayed, read psalms, and then burned incense and sprinkled holy water over the dying person. All that remained was to wait for death.

The ritual of dying, including the deathwatch which today is described by some people as a cruel, gruesome, and sadistic practice, was then accepted and carried out in a simple, ceremonial fashion. Although the ritual had elements of drama and the event undoubtedly aroused emotional feelings including fear, loss, guilt, and sorrow, there generally was no great show of emotion.

Several factors contributed to this simple acceptance. Death was familiar and expected. The recognition that death was imminent was not hidden either from the dying person or from anyone else, including children. Death occurred in bed in familiar surroundings, usually in the person's bedroom, which was *not* designated as a sick room; the dying person was fully aware that death was imminent. There was no expectation that death could be averted through medical therapies and consequently there were no attempts to try. The dying ritual was well known by all. It was expected and followed a pattern. It was shared in by family, friends, and neighbors. It was led by the dying person with the help of a priest or less frequently a physician. People did not die alone or separated from loved ones.

The belief in a common destiny prevailed during the early Middle Ages. The Christian view of death was accepted by nearly everyone: pious monk or knight or yeoman or peasant. The people of the early Middle Ages viewed dying and death as facts of life. They learned at a young age the behaviors which were to accompany dying and death. Dying and death were seen as a gateway to another life from which there was no escape and through which all must pass.

THE LATE MIDDLE AGES

Beginning around the eleventh and twelfth centuries a new Christian view emerged. Victory over death became less certain and visions of eternal torture gained prominence. Death was approached not only with less confidence but also with fear. There was a major preoccupation with death.

By the fourteenth century thoughts of eternal life brought little joy. Many people called themselves Christians but did not adhere to the tenets of Christianity. The Church assumed responsibility for reminding people of the warnings of the Gospels and of the need to prepare for the expected return of Christ or be doomed. It was a time of pentecostal processions designed to alert people to this day of reckoning. Emphasis was placed upon retribution rather than reward. The hereafter became a source of terror, not consolation, and a place of retribution, not reward (71).

10

In addition, during the late Middle Ages the fate of the individual became less bound with that of the community and a final judgment at the end of the world. Instead, the fate of the individual at the time of death and a judgment at the end of each life was stressed. Each person became responsible for his or her own destiny and, to a degree, that of others (72).

The change in emphasis was not without cost to the Christians. As Arnold Toynbee states: "when the belief in personal immortality is associated with a belief in judgment after death—a judgment that will consign the dead to either eternal bliss or eternal torment—the price of a human being's belief in the survival of his personality after death is anxiety during his lifetime (73)."

Many anxieties, or at least uncertainties, developed in relation to Christian reconciliation with the fact of death. These were related to the uncertainties of immortality and resurrection and to the prospect of eternal banishment and torture.

> The hereafter has become, through the efforts of the church, a source of terror and not consolation. Instead of reward, most people could expect only retribution. In order to secure a blissful existence in the other world, and not to be condemned eternally to unimaginable torture so vividly depicted by Hieronymus Bosch and others, it was necessary to lead such a life in this world as was beyond the endurance of most people, except for a few over-zealous ascetics. At the same time, as a result of the activity of priests and of monastic orders, an acute death consciousness became widespread. It is best expressed in the words, "Media in vita in morte sumus" (in the midst of life we are in death) (74).

Other factors contributed to keeping the fear of death alive. Kastenbaum and Aisenberg describe the fourteenth century as the crest of a period of uncontrollable and repulsive death. The late Middle Ages was a period characterized by warfare in which vicious brutalities were commonplace. Conditions were crowded, epidemics and pestilence ran unchecked, famine "strewed the roads with dead, and caused imprisoned thieves to devour one another (75)."

Bubonic plague occurred in various parts of Europe and was so terrible, malignant, and deadly that it brought its own special terrors. During plague times death was everywhere, stalking the streets.

There were no technological defenses, sanitation methods were unknown, even the disposal of bodies which littered the streets became a problem. Combining these horrendous social conditions with the view that death was God's punishment lent terror to death and made death the most dreaded moment of life.

Preoccupation with death was greater during the late Middle Ages than any other period in history. This preoccupation addressed the physical as well as the theological terrors associated with death (76).

Death was the favorite topic of preachers and moralists. The literature of the period described the agonies of death in a way that expressed the prevailing anxieties of the time but offered little in the way of consolation (77). The main theme of many of the paintings and woodcuts of the period was the "Triumph of Death," where Death was personified as the great equalizer.

Huizinga writes:

> . . . towards 1400 the conception of death in art and literature took a spectral

and fantastic shape. A new and vivid shudder was added to the great primitive horror of death. The macabre vision arose from deep psychological strata of fear; religious thought at once reduced it to a means of moral exhortation. As such it was a great cultural idea, til in its turn it went out of fashion lingering on in epitaphs and symbols in village cemeteries (78).

Although the horror of death was all-pervading and little reassurance was gained from the "mors melior vita" (death is better than life), death was *not* a tabooed subject in the late Middle Ages. It was quite the opposite as the fears and horrors of death were displayed openly. There was focus upon why death should be feared and no apologies were offered.*

The deathbed scene of the late Middle Ages was similar to that of the early Middle Ages in that the dying person followed the ritual in the presence of friends and relatives (79). However, there were important differences. Although the deathbed scene took place in the bedroom, the passive atmosphere of a waiting room changed to the more active clinical atmosphere of a sick room. In addition, the room was invaded by supernatural beings, who were representatives of "good" and "evil." It was believed that these representatives lined up on each side of the bed. There are many interpretations of this scene. Some interpret the scene as a battlefield, a contest between "good" and "evil" for the soul of the dying person who is the only witness to the event (80). Ariès (81) suggests another interpretation:

> God and His court are there to observe how the dying man conducts himself during this trial—a trial he must endure before he breathes his last and which will determine his fate in eternity. This test consists of a final temptation. The dying man will see his entire life as it is contained in the book, and he will be tempted either by despair over his sins, by "vainglory" of his good deeds, or by the passionate love for things and persons. His attitude during this fleeting moment will erase at once the sins of his life, if he wards off temptation, or on the contrary, will cancel out his good deeds if he gives way. The final test has replaced the Last Judgment.

Whatever the interpretation, the moment of death gained extreme impor-

---

* It would be fallacious to conclude that the doctrines which prevailed during the late Middle Ages were invented during the Middle Ages. T. Spencer, in *Death And Elizabethan Tragedy* (New York: Pageant Books, 1960, p. 3), writes of the philosophy of Plato "which taught that true reality lay outside the shadowy world of the senses, the metaphysical hierarchy of the neo-Platonists, which virtually identified evil with matter, the teaching of the stoics, who were compelled to face the worldly ills they did their best to deny, the visions of the Near-Eastern ascetics, who elaborated with increasing fervency of detail the tortures or delights of the next world—all these things made men look forward to death, and had prepared the way for a scorn of man's natural abilities and an emphasis on the next world which should be the only satisfactory attitude for serious minds to maintain. But Christianity added one remarkable doctrine which pagan disillusionment and transcendental philosophy had never mentioned. It taught that death was a punishment for man's sin." It is important to recognize that the doctrine of death as punishment for man's sin first appeared in the Old Testament and thus is a part of Judeo-Christian teachings.

tance. It had become the time of reckoning, the moment which gave the whole life meaning. With the belief that the dying person's attitude at the moment of death gave his whole life meaning, sudden death which provided no time for preparation was dreaded more than any other way of dying.

Despite the terrors associated with the moment of death during the late Middle Ages, the dying person remained the central figure. He knew what was expected in terms of his behavior. He presided over his death and directed the event as he wished. Death was accepted as inevitable, something that was always present within each individual. People recognized their own lifetime was a stay of execution. They were resigned to the fact that all people are mortal and will die. It is true that the degeneration of the body was seen as a sign of failure of the body, but it was not interpreted as a result of some personal failure, as in the twentieth century. Even though death held great horror for the people of the late Middle Ages, death was *not* a tabooed subject. People were resigned to the fact that death was unavoidable and inevitable. In fact, in the late Middle Ages death was the occasion which offered the greatest opportunity for development of self-awareness.

THE FIFTEENTH AND SIXTEENTH CENTURIES

Heightened concern with the process of dying in the late Middle Ages led to the development of a body of literature dealing with the art of dying. An English handbook called *The Craft of Dying* (82) (ca. 1450) is an example of an early volume written in the *ars moriendi* tradition. The tradition culminated in the seventeenth century with Jeremy Taylor's *The Rule and Exercises of Holy Dying* (83) (1651) which will be discussed later.

By the end of the fifteenth century death took on an erotic meaning. The art and literature of the period associated death with love, thanatos and eros. In addition, the Dance of Death theme—cavorting demons and skeletons leading men, women, and children down the paths to hell—became a predominant art theme. This theme was later seen in the works of such masters as Albrecht Dürer and Hans Holbein. The message was clear: death was the great equalizer, rich, poor, man, woman or child; none escaped. This fact could never be forgotten.

Death frequently was viewed as the grim reaper, the transgressor who tore people away from their daily lives. This concept of death as being snatched from life by an aggressive evil force was not seen earlier in history.

Ariès (84) suggested that the notion originated and was developed in the world of "erotic phantasms" and then passed "into the world of real and acted out events." It is difficult to evaluate whether death lost its erotic characteristics or whether they were sublimated. Whatever the explanation, although death was not desirable, it became admirable for its beauty. It became what was later to be called romantic death.

THE SEVENTEENTH THROUGH NINETEENTH CENTURIES

The seventeenth century heralded belief in a new meaning of death. Death was dramatized, exalted, and at the same time viewed as disruptive and greedy. There was a shift in focus from one's own death to the death of others.

13

The influence of science became more apparent during the eighteenth century than during any prior periods. This change in part is attributable to the philosophical climate associated with Descartes' conception of the mind and body as belonging to different orders of reality. The mind belonged to God and the supernatural and the body was of the natural world.

The separation of the supernatural orders of reality opened the way for rapid advances in the natural sciences. The scientific method was established as the theoretical matrix for understanding the natural world, including life and death, health and disease.

Men of medicine reflected the spirit of the sciences and adopted many of their methods, concepts, and ideas. There was a focus on healing and a search for the forces responsible for life. The prevailing thought appeared to be that understanding the forces *of* life might well provide the key *to* life.

There was a general waning of the view that disease, including disease of the mind, was attributable to demons, which was a popular conception in the sixteenth century. The physician was more and more called upon not only to treat but to cure ills.

Life and death became subjects for serious investigation. [Marie Francois] Xavier Bichat, a 28-year-old physician, published his *Vie et Mort* in 1800. The purpose of this daring book was to apply the tenets of scientific medicine in elucidating the nature of death itself. Bichat states (85): "Life and death, considered in a general manner, appeared to be a subject susceptible of several views and many useful experiments." He then proceeded to challenge the then traditional ideas about life and death by defining life as "the totality of those functions that resist death." He hypothesized two types of death, "natural death" and "accidental death." Natural death, the rarer of the two, was due to aging but could be accelerated by societal conditions such as overwork or poverty. Natural death was thought "to dim higher level mental functioning" and thus free the individual from death anxiety before "the lower level of visceral functioning was extinguished."

He attributed accidental death to body malfunction and performed a series of experiments to test the roles of the heart, brain, and lungs.

His book represents a turning point in modern Western ideas about mortality. It anticipates people's, more particularly the physician's, search for control over death. Bichat's organismic perspective formed the bridge to the scientific medicine of the nineteenth and twentieth centuries. Could scientific medicine provide the solution for the quest for eternal life? Could disease be conquered, health restored and thus could death not only be averted but conquered?

At the same time that medical and scientific questions were raised, other questions were addressed. The moral importance of the cirumstances under which a person died and the behavior the dying person displayed continued to be acknowledged during the seventeenth and eighteenth centuries. However, the then popular belief that "it did not matter how you lived so long as you died well," was seriously attacked by the spiritual writers of the period.

Jeremy Taylor, chaplain to King Charles the First, confronted death in *The Rule and Exercises of Holy Death* (86) (1651). Taylor was direct and uncompromising in his statements. He stated that "it is a great art to die well and to be learned by men in health, by them that can discourse and consider, by those whose understanding and acts of reason are not abated with fear or pains." He asserted that since the "greatest part of death is passed by the preceding years of our life," it was during those years that people should prepare for death, rather than during their last illness or on their deathbed. He advised that the "precepts of 'dying well' be a part of the studies of them that live in health." He urged daily examination of actions and behavior during health in preparation for actions and behavior at the deathbed. His comments on the benefits of the Church were pointed: ". . . it is not well that men should pretend anything will do a man good when he dies, and yet the same ministries . . . are found for forty or fifty years together to be ineffectual. . . . Can extreme unction at last cure what the holy sacrament of eucharist all his lifetime could not do?"

His insights are as useful today as when he wrote. He not only interwove the precepts of religion with the needs of dying people but also examined the fear of death and suggested ways to assist the dying person.

By the second half of the eighteenth century there was a major change in the prevailing relationship between the dying person and his or her family. Ariès (87) argued that the changes in wills reflected the changes in family relationships. It should be recalled that until the eighteenth century the focus primarily was upon the person threatened by death. From the thirteenth to the eighteenth century the last will and testament reflected just that. It was not simply a legal document for disposal of property. It was also a testament, a vehicle for expressing personal desires and thoughts about loved ones, religious beliefs, faith in God, personal possessions and salvation, and the cure and disposal of the body. It was written for the executor, the directors of the church, the curate of the parish, or the monks of the monastery and obligated them to carry out the wishes of the dead person. It imposed the dying person's will upon those around him, suggesting that he feared his wishes would not be listened to or obeyed. Generally, the will and testament took the place of face to face communication about these matters prior to death. Ariès suggested that the form of the will and testament reflected a distrust or at least indifference to the family. Of importance is the fact that the will and testament served the dying person. It assisted the person in managing her or his dying and the wants immediately following death.

By the second half of the eighteenth century the will became completely secularized.* It was reduced to the document which exists in contemporary society, a legal document designed to distribute fortunes according to the will of the deceased person. There are various explanations for this change. Vovelle (88) suggested that this secularization was one of the signs of the de-Christianization of society. Ariès proposed that the testament portion of the will was no longer necessary. By the end of the eighteenth century family relationships were based on feeling and affection; thus, the dying person expressed his views, feelings, and love for others orally. Until the end of the eighteenth century the dying person

---

*The importance of the roles of wills and testaments throughout history will become more apparent when discussing the twentieth century. As shall be seen, a new kind of will, the living will, was introduced in an attempt to restore to the dying person power over his fate. In addition, the testament portion of the secularized will was reintroduced as a personal means of sharing thoughts with loved ones.

commanded full power over the management of his dying. In trusting the next of kin, a part of the power was relinquished and delegated to the next of kin. The dying person still presided over his deathbed scene and continued to do so until the first few decades of the twentieth century. However, more and more power was relinquished to kin until the dying person no longer presided over the event nor, as shall be seen especially in the twentieth century, was he involved in decisions regarding his dying and death.

With the close of the eighteenth century came the end of a characteristically complacent attitude toward death and a conventional way of mourning. From the end of the Middle Ages until the end of the eighteenth century the level of mourning was controlled by social convention. It began after death, demanded appropriate manners and dress, and had specific duration.

The nineteenth century ushered in a period of exaggerated mourning which is reminiscent of the twelfth century. It was a period which contemporary psychologists might refer to as hysterical mourning.

Even though the deathbed scene of the nineteenth century was reminiscent of its ritual and its control by the dying person, there was a great difference. Although the dying individual presided over the solemn event surrounded by family and friends, the tone became openly emotional. Family and friends who were present wept, prayed aloud, fainted and shook with emotion. The demonstrative behavior persisted for an indeterminate duration. It might even reach a level of absurdity or madness with people joining in the delusional behavior of the mourner.

Another important change beginning in the eighteenth century and increasing in the nineteenth century was the renewed interest in tombs and cemeteries. Tombs and cemeteries, which did not play a predominant role during the Middle Ages, regained the place they had throughout antiquity. These new tombs did not contain the artifacts, iconography, and inscriptions of the ancient tombs such as the pyramids, but they did assure a kind of perpetuation. The memory of the dead conferred a kind of immortality for the individual, whereas the monuments became a symbol of the permanence of the society.

There are many ways to interpret this change. It might be suggested that the death of another person was no longer as easily accepted as in the past. It also might have reflected that the fear of death of another was as great or greater than the fear of one's own death. It might have been that the death of another evoked fears of self-vulnerability or perhaps the permanence of society itself was in question.

The need or desire for tombs and elaborate cemeteries suggested a lack of ease with the memories of the dead and a need for permanence. The art, literature, and spiritual issues suggested that people were troubled by the very thought of death. In short, the changes reflect the quandaries created by dying and death which were similar throughout Western civilizations.

During the course of the nineteenth century, however, differences in attitudes toward death evolved which can be identified in terms of clearly delineated geographic locations. These variations became especially apparent in the style and location of cemeteries and tombstones. The United States, England and parts of northwest Europe maintained the traditional simplicity of former periods. In addition, the commemorative monuments of heroes reflected a romantic concept of death. The commemorative monuments of American leaders, e.g., the Washington, Lincoln, and Jefferson memorials, are in keeping with this romantic concept. The Kennedy memorial especially reflects traditional simplicity. Continental Europe (France, Germany, and Italy) broke from this tradition. Cemeteries in those countries became extravagantly ornate.

There are various explanations given for these growing differences in practices which reflect attitudes toward death and dying. Some attribute the differences to religious orientations, that is, the Catholic mentality of continental Europe as contrasted to the Protestant view of England and North America. Although religion may have been one factor, its explanatory value is lessened when one considers that the separation of the churches occurred during the sixteenth century, approximately three centuries before there were any changes in burial practices (89).

Ariès explained the variations in attitudes toward death as a consequence of the socioeconomic revolution of the nineteenth century. He pointed out that extravagantly ornate funeral practices developed where economic growth was slow and where rural influences persisted such as they did in France, Italy, and Germany. In any case, the variation in attitudes between continental Europe and the United States and England increased. A general tolerance and acceptance of death persisted in continental Europe, whereas rapid socioeconomic advances in the United States contributed to a general abhorence of death, to the point of its becoming a "taboo" subject in the twentieth century.

REFERENCES

1. Benedict R: Patterns of Culture, New York, Houghton Mifflin Company, 1934, reprint ed., Mentor Books, New York, New American Library, 1946
2. Becker E: The Denial of Death, New York, The Free Press, 1973, pp. IX, 11 – 24; Feifel H: Religious conviction and fear of death among the healthy and terminally ill. *In* Fulton R (ed): Death and Identity, revised ed., Bowie, Md., The Charles Press Publishers, Inc., 1976, pp. 120 – 30; Weisman AD, Hackett TP: Predilection to death. *In* Fulton R (ed): Death and Identity, pp. 288 – 316; Kubler-Ross E: On Death and Dying, New York, The Macmillan Co., 1969, pp. 1 – 10; Wahl CW: The fear of death. *In* Fulton R (ed): Death and Identity, pp. 55 – 56
3. Dorr DI: Death. *In* Cargar H, White A (eds): Death and Hope, New York, Corpus Books, 1970, p. 7; Dumont RG, Foss DC: The American View of Death: Acceptance or Denial?, Cambridge, Mass., Schenkman Publishing Company, Inc., 1972, p. 1; McClelland DC: The harlequin complex. *In* White R (ed): The Study of Lives, New York, Atherton Press, 1963, p. 95
4. Feifel H: Death. *In* Faberow NL (ed): Taboo Topics, New York, Atherton Press, 1963, pp. 8 – 21; Carrington H: Death and Its Causes and Phenomena with Special Reference to Immortality, New York, Dodd, Mead and Co., Inc., 1921, p. 4
5. Choron J: Death and Western Thought, New York, Collier Books, 1963, p. 14
6. Levy-Bruhl L: Primitive Mentality, London, Allen and Unwin, 1923, pp. 37 – 38
7. For examples see Murdock G: Our Primitive Contemporaries, New York, Macmillan Co., 1934; Henderson JL, Oakes M: The Wisdom of the Serpent; The Myths of Death, Rebirth, and Resurrection, New York, Braziller, 1963
8. Choron, Death and Western Thought, p. 14

9. Riley JW, Jr.: Death and bereavement. *In* International Encyclopedia of the Social Sciences, 1968, pp. 4, 20
10. Radin P: Gott und Mensch in der Primitiven Welt, Zurich, Rhein Verlag, 1953, enlarged German edition of the *World of Primitive Man*, trans. Margaritta von Wyss, pp. 417 – 18
11. Choron, Death and Western Thought, pp. 15 – 16
12. Frazer Sir J: The Belief in Immortality, London, The Macmillan Company, 1913, p. 468
13. Murdock, Primitive Contemporaries, pp. 11, 17
14. Henderson, Oaks, Wisdom of the Serpent, p. 4
15. Murdock, Primitive Contemporaries, p. 215
16. Ducasse CJ: The Belief in Life after Death, Springfield, Ill., Charles C. Thomas, 1961, p. 290
17. Head J, Cranston SL, (eds): Reincarnation: The Phoenix Fire Mystery, New York, Julian Press/Crown Publishers, Inc., 1977,; Robak M (ed): A Handbook on Reincarnation, New York, Death Education Books, 1979
18. Agee J: A Death in the Family, New York, Avon Book Division, The Hearst Corporation, 1957, pp. 141 – 45; Dickens C: A Christmas Carol
19. Bernstein M: The Search for Bridey Murphy, New York, Doubleday, 1956, 1965; Holzer HW: Born Again, 1st ed., Garden City, New York, Doubleday, 1970
20. Harmer RM: The High Cost of Dying, New York, Collier Books, 1963, pp. 51, 55 – 56
21. Simmons L: The Role of the Aged in Primitive Society, New Haven, Yale University Press, 1948
22. The Book of the Dead, trans. Tirard HM, London, E.S. Gorham, 1910
23. Choron, Death and Western Thought, p. 22
24. Wilson A: The Culture of Ancient Egypt, Chicago, University of Chicago Press, 1956, p. 297
25. Hamilton E: The Greek Way, New York, Norton, 1930, p. 17
26. Lattimer R: Themes in Latin and Greek Epitaphs, Urbana, Ill., University of Chicago Press, 1962
27. Choron: Death and Western Thought, p. 80
28. Ruth JE: Toward a general theory of healing. unpubl. doctoral diss., The Hartford Seminary Foundation, 1975; Xerox University Microfilms, 1976, p. 53
29. Sirach 17:1 – 2 (NAB)
30. Sirach 14:17 – 18 (NAB)
31. 2 Samuel 14:14 (NAB)
32. Ecclesiastes 9:7, 10
33. Genesis 1:31 (NAB)
34. Genesis 3:14 – 19
35. Sirach 17:19 – 27 (NAB)
36. Isaiah 38:10 (NAB)
37. Psalms 102:25 (NAB)
38. Proverbs 5:21 – 23 (NAB)
39. Psalms 55:24 (NAB)
40. Job 4:7 – 9 (NAB). See also Job 8:8 – 20 (NAB)
41. Job 21:7 – 34 (NAB)
42. Job 1:21 (NAB)
43. Sirach 18:1 – 13 (NAB)
44. Isaiah 25:8 (NAB)
45. Isaiah 26:19 (NAB)
46. Daniel 12:2 (NAB)

47. Job 19:25 — 27 (NAB)
48. Abbott WM, Gilbert A, Hunt R, Swain J: The Bible Reader: An Interfaith Interpretation, New York, The Bruce Publishing Company, 1969, p. 600 (For explicit statements regarding immortality see Wisdom 3:5; 5:15; 15:3 (NAB)
49. Abbott, Bible Reader, p. 597
50. Wisdom 3:5 (NAB)
51. Abbott, Bible Reader, p. 597
52. Micah 6:8 (NAB)
53. 1 Corinthians 15:51 — 57 (NAB)
54. Choron, Death and Western Thought, p. 85
55. Choron, Death and Western Thought, p. 85
56. Isaiah 25:8 — 9
57. John 14:1 — 7; Matthew 5:12 (NAB)
58. Romans 5:12 — 15 (NAB)
59. Romans 6:9 (NAB)
60. 1 Corinthians 15:22 (NAB)
61. Romans 6:1 — 11 (NAB)
62. 1 Corinthians 15:12 — 28 (NAB)
63. Acts 17:31 — 32 (NAB)
64. 1 Thessalonians 4:13 — 18 (NAB); see also 1 Corinthians 15:35 — 44
65. John 3:16 (NAB)
66. John 15:13
67. 2 Corinthians 5:18
68. Matthew 5:12 (NAB)
69. Dorr, in Death and Hope, pp. 8 — 11
70. Mark 13:24 — 37; Matthew 25:31 — 56; Luke 17:22 — 37 (NAB)
71. Choron, Death and Western Thought, p. 91
72. Dorr, in Death and Hope, pp. 7 — 11
73. Toynbee A: Various ways in which human beings have sought to reconcile themselves to the fact of death. In Schneidman ES (ed): Death: Current Perspectives, Palo Alto, Calif., Mayfield Publishing Co., 1976, p. 37
74. Choron, Death and Western Thought, p. 91
75. Kastenbaum R, Aisenberg R: Psychology of Death, New York, Springer Publishing Co., Inc., 1972, p. 195
76. Spencer T: Death and Elizabethan Tragedy, New York, Pageant Books, 1960, p. 11
77. Spencer, Death and Elizabethan Tragedy, p. 11
78. Huizinga J: The Waning of the Middle Ages: A Study of Life, Thought and Art in France and the Netherlands in the XIVth and XVth Centuries, Garden City, New York, Doubleday Anchor Books, 1963, p. 144
79. Ariès P: Western Attitudes Toward Death From the Middle Ages to the Present, trans. Ranum PM, Baltimore, The Johns Hopkins University Press, 1974, p. 34
80. Choron, Death and Western Thought, p. 92
81. Ariès, Western Attitudes Toward Death, p. 92
82. Comper, FMM (ed): The Book of the Craft of Dying and Other Early English Tracts Concerning Death. Taken from manuscripts and printed books in the British Museum and Bodleian Libraries with preface by the Rev. George Congreve (N.B.).
83. Taylor J: The Rule and Exercises of Holy Dying, Boston, Little, Brown and Company, 1864; also see Taylor J: Holy Living and Dying: With Prayers Containing the Whole Duty of a Christian, and Parts of Devotion Fitted to All Occasions and For All Necessities, London, G. Bell Sons, 1913

84. Ariès, Western Attitudes, p. 63
85. Bichat [MF] X: Physiological Researches Upon Life and Death, trans. from French by Tobias Watkins, First American Form, Second Paris ed., Philadelphia, Smith and Maxwell, 1809, p. IX
86. Taylor, Rule and Exercises of Holy Dying, pp. IX – X
87. Ariès, Western Attitudes, p. 63
88. Vovelle M: Piete baroque et dechristianisation, Paris 1973, as cited in Ariès, Western Attitudes, p. 64
89. Ariès, Western Attitudes, p. 80

2   The Twentieth Century: Death—a Social Problem

P rior to the turn of the twentieth century, views of life and death in the United States were like those of other Western nations. During the seventeenth through nineteenth centuries Americans perceived a continuity between life and death. They saw life as a preparation for death. Thus, life *and* death were viewed as integral parts of the human experience. The reality of death was recognized and accepted. Mortality rates were high; deaths were witnessed frequently and directly. Epidemics were common as were deaths in infancy and early childhood. There were few families who did not lose a family member at a young age; but people were not morbidly preoccupied with death as they were during the late Middle Ages. There were no art forms depicting the dance of death nor were there books on the art of dying. There was a commitment to work and a striving to improve one's quality of life. For some, success in life predicted success in life after death. For others, hardships during life earned rewards in an afterlife. Thus, there was a sense of control over the power of death.

Dying individuals continued to preside over their own deaths. The death-watch was maintained. Death occurred at home with family, friends, and children in attendance. It was a sad and usually unwelcomed event and, yet, it was not seen as something separate from life, something tabooed and unmanageable both for the individual and for society.

DEATH: UNMANAGEABLE AND TABOO

Many interrelated factors contributed to the growing view of death as a catastrophe and to the rapidly changing attitudes related to life and to death. These changes contributed to making death virtually unmanageable for twentieth century American society and for individuals dying in that society. These factors are related to the tenor of the times and to the ageless, universal need to believe that death is not the absolute end and that survival after death is not an illusion. In addition, these factors are associated with the desire to believe there is significance to and beyond each individual life. Therefore, death is controllable and man immortal.

In general, the 1900's marked a period of rapid social change. They were a time of unprecedented technological advances, an age of great medical accomplishments, and a period of great expansion and industrialization. During the 1900's there was also serious questioning of values and institutions; it was a time of massive violence and death. Of greater relevance, there was much searching for the meaning of life and avoidance of the consideration of death.

TWO REALMS: LIFE AND DEATH

The early twentieth century gave rise to remarkable changes in views toward life and toward death. The most apparent change was the growing conception of life and death as two distinct entities. Life was vested with meaning and death was seen more and more as meaningless and irrelevant. Death, once again, became viewed as a transgressor and a usurper of life. Moreover, death became an enemy to be conquered.

Irion (1) attributes the breach in continuity between life and death to the deism of the eighteenth century, to the increasing acceptance of humanism, and to the world view of modern science. He contends that the view of death as part of life is contradictory to some of the major expectations of American life. For example, because Americans conquered the frontiers, they assume that it is just a matter of time before they can overcome all obstacles. Whether the focus is knowledge, freedom, or possessions, Americans believe they can be conquered. In much current thought this conquering phenomenon, which Irion calls "expansion," represents progress. He argues that since death cannot be eliminated, it represents an impediment to life, and as such is not a part of life.

Materialism is another factor which contributes to the American view of death as something separate from life. When there is a focus upon the value of material elements of life, then death becomes a destroyer. The very thought of death is antithetic to life. Believing that progress includes accumulation of material wealth and expansion of frontiers, Americans will not accept anything that seems to negate this belief. Death is viewed as negative, therefore it is separated from life. Persons holding these views avoid thinking about and talking about their own deaths and they attempt to divert thoughts of dying from those who are facing death.

Wahl (2) discusses the relationship between the emphasis upon progress and the definition of death as a catastrophe. He suggests that twentieth century Americans pride themselves on their ability to control their physical and social environments such as by flying to the moon or by treating once incurable ills. Yet, although scientists may be able to delay death and sometimes to decrease the miseries of dying, they cannot eliminate it. Thus, death is intrusive and perplexing—a catastrophic event.

It might be inferred that death, then, is something which happens *to* life and therefore is not a part *of* life. Since death is inevitable, the thought of death or the sight of death increases anxiety and fear and thus increases the need to deny and to avoid death or even the mention of death on the one hand, and to eliminate or at least to control death on the other.

DEATHS: MASSIVE YET UNWITNESSED

Although Americans have not yet succeeded in their attempt to eliminate death, they have succeeded in creating the illusion of controlling death through modern weaponry (e.g., atomic, cobalt, and hydrogen bombs). These weapons not only cause the deaths of individuals, but can destroy total populations. In addition, they increase the fear of violent and catastrophic death. The deaths of millions of people in wars and extermination camps is the legacy of the twentieth century.

Ironically, at the same time that death is seen as an enemy and not a part of life, the destruction of the world has become a reality. Armageddon has become a possible consequence of man's decision, not the consequence of the will of God, nor of the laws of nature (3).

Although millions of people have been killed in war and catastrophes, most Americans keep distant from the reality of death. The average American experiences death in his family only once in every twenty years (4). Most of these deaths occur in hospitals, nursing homes, homes for the aged, or like institutions. Many times family members are not present and the person dies alone or in the presence of strangers. People no longer witness the whole cycle of life. In fact, many people have witnessed neither the birth of a baby nor the death of another human being.

There was a time when deaths were experienced directly and the sight of death was common. People died in their own homes surrounded by their families. Several generations lived in the same house and the life cycle was seen as a whole. Birth, growth, health, sickness, and death were seen as part of the human experience.

Seeing someone die is not sufficient to relieve the tensions associated with dying and death. Authors (5) have demonstrated that witnessing dying and death does not necessarily lead to increased options of behavior for either dying persons or those interacting with them. Many physicians and nurses who witness dying and death exhibit the same avoidance behavior as lay people when interacting with dying persons (6). This avoidance behavior includes limiting interactions with the dying person, avoiding conversations about the status of the person's health, and focusing upon physical components of care and scientific explanations of expected positive effects of current therapies. What, then, are the implications of not witnessing death directly, yet hearing of the deaths of many in a society in which death is not generally seen as a part of life?

Kubler-Ross (7) contends that the news of large numbers of people killed in war and on the highway allows people to conceive of the deaths of others and not their own. Such news not only supports peoples' unconscious belief in immortality, but it also allows them to rejoice that it is not they but other people who die.

CERTAIN DEATH AND IMMORTALITY

The news of massive deaths coupled with the twentieth century emphasis on scientific control and explanation has dispelled the age-old myth of death as a chance event, an accident, something that happens to someone else. It has also reinforced the recognition of death as a certainty for all.

The *wish* to perceive death as a chance event and as something that happens to others persists. People now, as in the past, simultaneously recognize death as inevitable and, yet, maintain belief in their own immortality.

The phenomenon of recognizing the reality of death while preserving a belief in immortality was addressed by Freud (8) in *Thoughts for the Times on War and Death*, written shortly after the beginning of World War I. Freud believed that people have a fundamental inability to imagine their own death. Yet, at the same time, conscious attitudes are changed by feelings of helplessness and lack of control engendered by the actual occurrence of many deaths and by recognizing that death is inevitable. People can think about their own deaths yet they cannot consider their total annihilation. People cannot imagine the actual end of their lives on earth. The fact that people can continue to think about other persons who have died causes them to conceive of a continuity beyond death.

Freud's concept of "unconscious immortality" is reminiscent of the primitive view that people would live forever were it not for accidents, magic, or mystical forces. If life has to end, then the ending must be attributed to a malicious intervention by someone or something outside of the individual. A person can be killed, but it is inconceivable that one can die of something inherent, such as aging. (Nobody ever dies of old age.) As a result, death is a frightening happening, something associated with a malicious act which calls for retribution (9).

Death has also become something that can be controlled by scientific means. There is a growing body of literature exploring the possibility of extending the vigorous years of life for many years, perhaps forever. Rosenfeld asks in his book *Prolongevity* (10), "Can we live to be 150? 200?" He offers an optimistic response: "Eventually we will harness DNA and its genetic code to our own ends. When we begin to do that . . . we will be on our way to the final quest of old age," and it might be inferred to the quest of death.

"Death is an imposition on the human race, and no longer acceptable" declares Harrington in *The Immortalist* (11). Although such a statement may be interpreted in many ways, it seems reasonable to infer that poor judgment, or lack of care, is to blame if death occurs. Thus, but for poor judgment or lack of care, people could live forever.

So strong is the unconscious belief in immortality, that studies of survivors of atomic bombings or extermination camps attest that the belief persists, even when whole populations are confronted with imminent death (12). Persistence of this belief is seen in the statement by Joe Barauch, a Vietnam war veteran: "I was becoming impervious to the death of my fellow soldiers, and in addition, I was negating the possibility of my own possible demise." (13)

Experiencing uncontrollable death does not alone lead to treating death as a tabooed event. As previously discussed, uncontrollable deaths of the late Middle Ages contributed to a morbid preoccupation with the spectacle of death, as well as to an emphasis upon openly proclaiming the horrors of death and the reasons to fear death. In contrast to the twentieth century, however, during the late Middle Ages, death was viewed not only as an inevitable event but as an integral part of life. In addition, dying people and those interacting with them knew what behavior was expected of them. The dying person was expected to preside over his or her dying. He or she was not stripped of power over the situation. He or she was not expected to wage war with death. Death was not perceived as meaningless, nor was it expected that death could be conquered by human intervention. Death was seen as the event which offered the opportunity for an individual to develop self-awareness.

In fact, in the age of the Dance of Death, the physician was rarely depicted in woodcuts or other art forms (14). The physician, when pictured, was shown as an impotent mortal, the main butt of the jokes of the skeleton of death. The picture of the physician as a foe of death and a fighter against clinical disease did not appear until the concepts of clinical illness and clinical death were developed and generally accepted (15).

DEATH: NEEDLESS AND PREMATURE

Although the relinquishing of dying persons' power to preside over their own deaths began following World War I, it was not generally apparent until shortly after World War II. The dying *person* gradually became the dying *patient*. The physician rather than the dying person struggled with death and death reflected the physician's failure to win the battle with death.

As in primitive societies, someone or something external to the individual could be blamed when death triumphed. However, unlike primitive societies, the enemy was not limited to the physician or any one person. Society was indicted. It was the injustices of society which deprived working-class people of appropriate medical attention and care. Society and the medical profession were indicted for changes in medical care including the practice of refusing to make house calls. The concept of "clinical death" became well entrenched. People no longer died of natural causes; instead, there was a host of specific etiologies for their clinical demise (16). Deaths became clinically avoidable and thus premature. For every premature or clinically unnecessary death, Illich argued, somebody could be found who irresponsibly delayed or prevented medical attention. "Clinical death" reflected the belief that but for the lack of medical attention, all would survive. As a consequence, most, if not all, deaths could be interpreted as clinically avoidable or unnecessary and premature.

This view of death as clinically unnecessary created problems for all, but especially for the survivors. It evoked feelings of guilt or anger, as well as the need for self-punishment, retribution, reevaluation of prior decisions, actions, or professional expertise, depending upon the individual's role in the situation. These problems and dilemmas were compounded when death was perceived as premature. The thought of someone being "struck down in the prime of life" has always aroused fear and consternation. What is unique to the twentieth century, however, is that regardless of a person's age or attendant circumstances, death is usually seen as premature. If there is not a belief in some continuity between life and death and in some significance beyond the life of one individual, death becomes meaningless, uncontrollable, unacceptable and profoundly threatening. There is thus a need to avoid death, deny its existence, or treat it as an abnormal event distinct from life.

Illich believes that death has become a metaphorical figure and that the killer diseases have taken its place. The physician is expected to do battle with disease and to have the power to control the outcome of disease. Some people, physicians and lay people alike, have extended this belief to include a power over life and death.

Following World War II, many factors contributed to the development, continuation, and expansion of the myth of the physician's power over death. Major discoveries and advances were made in science and in medicine. Use of antibiotics all but eliminated or rendered impotent major infectious diseases such as pneumonia. Advances in anesthesia made new and daring surgeries possible.

There was increased professional and societal recognition of the need for better prepared physician specialists,* followed by the recognition of the need for better prepared nurses, social workers, and dentists. As technology increased, new technicians and paraprofessionals developed.

At the same time these changes were occurring in medicine and science, changes were occurring in society. Social security benefits became a reality and coverage for medical care became part of union contracts. There was a demand for continuing health care after retirement. People not only planned to retire, but they expected to live a comfortable, healthy, and productive life. Health care became viewed as a right of all people and not a privilege for a few. Society became responsible for preventing death. Medical treatment, effective or not, became mandatory. If people died, it was expected that it occurred while they were receiving care from clinically competent care providers. Even then, some people were skeptical as to whether death was necessary. There were changes in the nature of dying brought about by advances in modern medicine and technology.

CHANGES IN THE NATURE OF DYING

Death has changed; it is no longer as likely to be sudden. The pattern of illness and death has shifted from acute infectious diseases to chronic conditions. There is usually a period of illness preceding death. This pattern is true for the young who experience catastrophic illnesses such as some forms of cancer, autoimmune disease, or cardiovascular disease, as it is true for the aged.

There are predicted survival rates accompanying many diagnoses and types of medical therapies. Health care professionals and lay people alike are aware of the morbidity and mortality patterns associated with survival rates. A patient once asked, "I'm glad my cancer was operable, but when do you start counting the five years [survival rate]?"

In a society which views life and death as separate entities, the period of life or living after the diagnosis of a usually fatal illness is often seen as part of dying rather than as part of living. Many problems, as well as many legal and ethical questions and issues, arise during this period of living when a person is actively or recognizably dying.

Medical and scientific advances have contributed to the problems and dilemmas associated with dying and they have given rise to many questions. Who shall be kept alive? For how long? For what purposes? And by what means? What are the criteria for death? Who has, or what is, the right to die? Who should have the responsibility or authority for discontinuing extraordinary means of maintaining life? What is the definition of extraordinary means? Modern medicine and technology have become so sophisticated it now is difficult to know when dying and not living is being prolonged.

---

*For a complete discussion of the changes in medicine and the role of the physician, see Richard H. Shryock, The Development of Modern Medicine: An Interpretation of the Social and Scientific Factors Involved, New York, Alfred A. Knopf, Inc., 1947.

QUALITY IN LIVING: DIGNITY IN DYING

By the late 1960's and early 1970's more explicit emphasis was being placed upon quality of life rather than focusing solely on length of life (17). There was an increasing consideration of consumer's rights and there was controversy over the growing belief that it is beneficial to have open discussions about dying and death. In addition, there was work on methods to identify and assure the rights of dying people (18).

DYING PATIENT'S BILL OF RIGHTS

One method for assuring the rights of the dying was the introduction of the Dying Patient's Bill of Rights (19). Although these statements were not widely distributed or publicized, they were intended to offer guidelines to dying people and to those caring for them. The intent was to provide dying people information so that they might participate in making informed decisions regarding their care for as long as they were able. Although various interest groups developed different forms, most addressed as the primary right the right of patients to be informed about the gravity of their illness and the likelihood of their death. Other rights included the right to die with dignity unencumbered by tubes and machines in an atmosphere of hopefulness, surrounded by loved ones instead of strangers no matter how highly skilled. The right to privacy. The right to receive care from sensitive, knowledgable, caring persons who attempt to understand the patient's needs and the needs of the families and friends.

LIVING WILLS

Concern over the powerlessness of dying persons and their rights, especially the right to die with dignity, led to the development of the living will (20). The living will is a document directed to the person's family, lawyer, clergy, physician, or other responsible persons. These wills cover situations where a person is no longer able to make decisions about his or her future or when there is no reasonable expectation for recovery. In general, living wills request that the individual be allowed to die with dignity and not be kept alive by extraordinary means. Some living wills request that medications be administered to alleviate pain and suffering even though it may hasten the moment of death. The intent of the request is not for euthanasia, but for comfort and quality of life until death.

Living wills are not legally binding in all states and many questions continue to be raised about the conditions under which they could or should be honored. There is growing demand, however, for their use and legislation to support them is underway in some states.

THE HOSPICE MOVEMENT

Another significant development demonstrating the importance of and concern for restoring dignity and power to dying persons is the growth of the hospice movement. Hospice, a familiar term in medieval times, described a place of comfort and hospitality. Hospices were characterized by a sense of community and an atmosphere of caring. Usually under the sponsorship of religious orders, hospices were places of refuge for weary pilgrims and other travelers.

Today, the word hospice is not used to mean only a place or a particular building, but it is a *concept* of *health care* for dying people and their families. Hospice care can be accomplished in a person's home as well as in specially designed buildings, or in specially designed or designated parts of an existing hospital.

Hospice has come to mean a health care program offering continuous supportive care to dying people and significant others.* This program enables people to live out the final days of their lives as comfortably and as fully as possible. The complete concept of hospice includes a family approach in caring for terminally ill people 24 hours a day, seven days a week in their homes, or in a special inpatient facility. It includes a bereavement program for family and other closely involved individuals which lasts for one year following the death of their loved one. Those who wish to may participate longer. The concept also includes educational programs for dying persons, their families, significant others, volunteers, and health care professionals.

Admission to an inpatient hospice is determined by the needs of dying persons and their families. Individuals may be admitted to establish a pain control program, or because family members are unable to cope with care. Admissions may be short-term or permanent. In either case, family members are encouraged to be present and to participate in care.

The overall purpose of hospice care is to promote quality of living for terminally ill persons and their families. The objective is to assist dying persons and their families to face death with minimal pain and fear. Hospice care attempts to free the terminally ill from pain and suffering and to maintain their quality of life. Medical and nursing interventions are reasonable, not heroic, and are directed at preventing symptoms and thus alleviating some of the fears associated with dying. In addition, terminally ill persons and their families are assisted to live with dying in a pleasant family-centered environment.

Discussions of how, where, and by whom the hospice concept of care should be implemented are beyond the province of this book. Those readers who wish to learn more about hospice should see reference 21. Even a cursory overview of the hospice movement, however, reflects a new awareness and recognition of death as inevitable and acceptable in American society. Even so, it is premature to characterize it as the predominant view of dying and death today. There are other views that are variations of two distinct and, at times, almost antithetical trends.

One is the movement toward restoring the concept of continuity between life and death by bringing death into the open and dealing with it as a part of living. This view may include some concept of a life after death either based upon religious tenets or rational secular views of life after this life (22). The other view negates the inevitability of death, treats it as an enemy and hides it as though it were a failure or an embarrassing family secret. Usually, this view is manifested by avoiding the mention of death and by avoiding other interactions with the dying person.

---

*Significant others refers to people important to the dying person, such as friends, associates, and relatives other than the immediate family. Family refers to the immediate family members.

THE TRADITION OF SECRECY

Avoidance of the topic of dying and the avoidance behavior observed in those interacting with dying persons are examples of a broader cultural pattern—the tradition of secrecy. The tradition of secrecy is characterized by patterned and accepted avoidance and includes the development of stable, patterned behaviors and relationships with rules and a system of sanctions and rewards. Such a tradition of secrecy, whether by chance or planned intent, prevents learning from various situations from taking place.

In some respects, confidentiality can be considered a tradition of secrecy. Although there is no question that confidentiality is important and necessary in some situations, the paramount question is when and how much confidentiality is necessary and functional for society. The maintenance or expansion of realms of secrecy and confidentiality, for whatever reason, may lead to dysfunctional consequences by eliminating the opportunity to learn from a situation and to develop competencies in interaction with the situation.

When these interactions are not open to or available for observation and scrutiny, society at large is denied the opportunity to learn the essential components of the interaction. How can we help people facing terminal illness if we know so little about the thoughts and behaviors of individuals facing imminent death, or if we do not understand the social situation and interactions surrounding the dying person?

Blumer (23) proposes that the empirical social world is the world of everyday experiences and that we learn from observing and participating in a situation by observing and interviewing those involved. We can expect, therefore, to gain understanding of the social situation of dying persons and the social processes surrounding them by studying their empirical world.

RESEARCH ON DYING AND DEATH

Although fear of death was recognized as a researchable subject as early as 1896 (24), relatively little study of the fear of dying and death was conducted prior to 1950 (25). Suicide, war, disaster, and accidents as modes of death received considerably more attention from social scientists than death under more natural circumstances (26).

There are several explanations for the disproportionate attention given to unnatural deaths. Investigators may have had greater access to mortality data derived from statistical rather than from first-hand field experiences. Investigators perhaps perceived use of statistical data as decreasing their dependence upon beliefs, values, or attitudes of others. The fact that these deaths, theoretically at least, might be prevented or at least reduced in numbers, may have provided a special incentive and challenge to researchers and their sponsors. Whatever the reason, the social scientist who works solely with statistical data is removed from direct experience with dying and death.

These studies themselves reflect the realities of the empirical world which they attempt to explain. They suggest that often the researcher's own aversions may stand in the way of doing social psychological studies of dying and death. The perceptions and feelings of the investigators are as important as the reactions and feelings of those who are dying. This is clearly shown as Keen (27) described his reactions to his deathbed interview with Ernest Becker.

He said that he felt it presumptuous to intrude upon the private world of the dying person. Keen considered it even more presumptuous, however, not to respond to the invitation of this dying philosopher. The interview would not have been attempted if Becker had not insisted. Moreover, even as the interview was being conducted, Keen was still troubled by his own preconceived notions. He stated:

> Our conversation started slowly. I asked leading questions and Becker answered. At times my mind raised objections but I did not have the heart to push critical points. The hours wove us together and our talk became crisper. It was clear that Becker neither wanted nor offered intellectual quarter.

STUDIES OF PERSONS FACING IMMINENT DEATH*

Feifel (28) was one of the first investigators to emphasize the importance of studying death by talking with dying people. He encountered many difficulties in gaining the support of physicians and administrators who interpreted discussing death with seriously or terminally ill people as cruel, sadistic, and traumatic. Their interpretations differed, however, from that of those who were dying. Patients expressed to Feifel the desire to be informed about their conditions and felt that discussing their illnesses helped them to adjust to the experience of dying. His findings suggest that dying individuals may define the situation differently than those responsible for their care.

Kubler-Ross (29), a psychiatrist, experienced the same professional barriers when she sought entry to dying people. She asked the patients to be her teacher so that she might learn more about the final stages of life with all its fears, anxieties, and hopes.

Patients responded to her with amazement that anyone would want to spend time listening to them and gratitude at having been heard. Their surprise may have reflected their awareness of the generally taboo nature of the topic and their recognition that such discussion breaks a commonly accepted rule of behavior, the avoidance of subject matter which may cause discomfort to others. As Kubler-Ross described it, the initial outcome in the majority of cases was similar to opening floodgates. She had difficulty stopping them once conversation was initiated. The "patients responded with great relief to sharing their last concerns, expressing their feelings without fear of repercussions."

Kubler-Ross did not have prior information regarding the patients' awareness of the seriousness of their conditions; she found this information irrelevant. After interviewing hundreds of terminally ill patients, she learned that they all were aware of the seriousness of their illness, whether they had been told explicitly or not. The patients informed Kubler-Ross, not vice versa.

---

*Although there are many important studies dealing with various aspects of dying and death (e.g., attitudes, fears, bereavement), this section will focus solely upon selected studies of dying people.

Patients who were told directly of the seriousness of their illnesses almost unanimously expressed their appreciation at having been informed. The exceptions were those patients who were told crudely: in corridors, without any preparation or follow-up, or in a fashion which left them without hope. Those patients who were not directly told the seriousness of their conditions gained their awareness from the implicit messages and altered behavior of relatives and health care providers. Glaser and Straus (30) similarly reported that many physicians and nurses believe that patients eventually learn that death is imminent, whether or not they are informed explicitly.

Kalish (31) has listed the following informational sources about their health available to patients: (1) direct statements from the physician; (2) overheard comments between health care providers; (3) direct statements from family, friends, lawyers, and hospital personnel including nursing personnel, technologists, other therapists; (4) changes in medical care routines, procedures, and medications; (5) changes in physical location; (5) reading materials—medical books, records, charts; and (7) changes in physical condition.

It is important to note, however, that even when patients were aware of their fate, they did not necessarily share their knowledge with their family and friends, or with health care providers. Although patients expressed to Kubler-Ross their desire to share their feelings of anger, rage, guilt, envy, and isolation, they "used denial" when they perceived that "denial" was expected by their physician or family members (32). They felt a need to share their concerns about impending death but shared them only with those they believed would take them seriously and would share their inner turmoil.

The observation that patients share their concerns with people whom they interpret as taking them seriously and understanding their situation demonstrates the importance of arriving at a consensus about the patient's situation. Once the people in the situation acknowledge agreement on the interpretation of the situation, the way is open for communication and interaction. Kubler-Ross invited patients to talk about dying, usually a taboo subject. In encouraging the discussion, she also established her recognition of the patient's awareness of the situation and created a common ground for interaction.

STAGES OR PHASES OF DYING

In *On Death and Dying* (33), Kubler-Ross used as an organizational scheme a series of stages through which most people pass in response to their awareness of dying.

Regardless of how people became aware of the terminal nature of their illness, they reacted to the news in the same way human beings react to any great and unexpected stress—namely, with shock and disbelief. This initial reaction was followed by a stage of denial and isolation, a "no, not me, it cannot be true" response. Denial gave way to a second stage, anger, "why me?" This was followed by a temporary stage called bargaining, the attempt to postpone dying, with the bargaining stage ending in depression. Depression was the "stepping stone" to the final stage, acceptance. All people maintained hope in some form. In Kubler-Ross's view, it did not matter what the stage or the way people discovered that death was imminent.

Careful reading of Kubler-Ross suggests that she did not intend these stages to represent a concrete and specific sequential series of stages through which a dying person *must* pass. Rather, she cites illustrations where these stages did not occur; however, some of her followers interpreted these stages as absolutes. Unfortunately, these absolutes were interpreted as: if the patients are to die well, they must pass through all these stages sequentially.

Following the publication of *On Death and Dying*, there was a surge of literature which referred to the stages of dying and the importance of open communication about dying with dying people. The goal of many health care providers became that of assisting dying patients through the stages so they might die a "good" death. Some health care providers believed they were responsible for assisting dying persons through the stages and that these persons were obligated to progress through the stages.

The consequences of this rigid interpretation and application were not always positive. The use of the stages imposed their own constraints upon the behavior of patients, family members, and health care providers. The author has talked with nurses who reported becoming angry at patients who did not progress through the stages as expected. They expressed feelings of failing professionally for not being able to assist patients to fit this pattern. Many health care personnel, family members, and patients familiar with the stages interpreted passing through the stages as "the right way to die," the "scientific way to die;" no other way was acceptable. There was a way to die, and that way was not perceived as related to the way the person had lived or chose to die.

Questions about the accuracy and usefulness of "the stages of dying" for patients or those helping them began to be addressed. In 1974, Weisman (34) examined the concept of stages through use of a method called the "psychological autopsy" which reconstructs the psychological process of dying. He identified no well-recognized succession of emotional responses that are typical of people facing imminent death. Further, he described "the idea of staging [as] very artificial." He suggested that there might be "phases" rather than "stages" of dying.

The findings of Schultz and Aderman (35) support those of Weisman. They did not find that patients go through stages, but that they adopt a pattern of behavior and that pattern persists until death. Another investigator, Shibles (36), evaluated the Kubler-Ross stages as being "too procrustean, narrow, or fixed."

Three phases of dying, "acute," "chronic living-dying," and "terminal," were proposed by Pattison (37) who cautioned that these phases were only a convenient way of dividing the living-dying process for clinical utility and increased understanding of the behaviors accompanying dying.

Kubler-Ross's work contributed toward breaking the conspiracy of silence about dying and death. Investigators began studying various problems and factors related to dying.

AWARENESS CONTEXTS AND DYING TRAJECTORIES

The problem of awareness as a salient factor in interactions was the focus of Glaser and Strauss (38). They reported that the interactions between dying people and others are guided by each person's awareness of the dying state.

They identified four commonly occurring situations which they referred to as *awareness contexts*. These ranged from *closed awareness* to *total awareness*. In *closed awareness* the patient does not recognize his or her impending death even though others have this information. In *total awareness* both the patient and others define him or her as dying, are aware of each other's definition, and are relatively open in their discussion of the patient's dying.

Glaser and Strauss also suggest five structural conditions which contribute to the existence of closed awareness: (1) Most patients are not especially experienced at recognizing the signs of impending death; (2) American physicians do not tell patients outright that death is probable or inevitable; (3) family members tend to guard as a secret that death is inevitable; (4) hospitals are arranged by accident or design to hide medical information from patients; and (5) patients have no allies who reveal or help them discover the staff's knowledge of their impending death. In spite of these factors, Glaser and Strauss found that health professionals commonly held the notion that patients should initiate the request for information regarding their health status.

Since Glaser and Strauss first published their study in 1964, there has been an upsurge of literature describing and analyzing dying, death, mourning, and bereavement (39). Many articles and books dealing with dying and death and with personal experiences with illnesses culminating in death are directed toward lay people (40). In addition, television programs and newspaper articles discuss various types of cancers and treatments, providing the public greater access to information about diagnostic labels frequently associated with dying. Depending upon individual circumstances and interpretations, this information may help or deter persons from arriving at a consensus about the situation.

In their later work, Glaser and Strauss (41) described the *status passage* involved in dying. *Status passage* refers to a fundamental change in a person's position in society which produces appreciable changes in relationships with others. The most familiar of these status passages are graduation from school, marriage, retirement, an election to a prominent office. Glaser and Strauss refer to the transition from life (being) to death (non-being) as an unwelcomed status passage. In describing the status passage or courses of dying, they use the term *dying trajectories*. According to them, expectations of death are key determinants in how patients and those interacting with them act during the course of dying.

They also suggest transitional stages within the passage from living to dying (42). They refer to these as *transitional statuses*. Because their categories are based upon the distinctions medical personnel make in viewing death expectations, it is more a typology than a continuum. It may be, however, that under varying conditions, the timing of the label may differ. The question may be raised: what conditions are present when people define themselves as dying or when others define them as dying?

Glaser and Strauss' first category refers to instances where there is question as to whether the individual will live or die, and health care personnel are unable to predict when the question will be resolved. For example, the person's physical status is tentative and there is little information regarding the effectiveness of alternative treatments. The second possibility is that there is uncertainty about death, but there is a known time when the question will be answered; such as, "We will know in 24 hours," or "The patient may or may not die; we will know after this surgery or treatment." The third is when death is inevitable, but the exact time it will occur cannot be predicted. The last category is when death is certain and the time of death can be predicted.

Some questions not considered by Glaser and Strauss are relevant for our understanding. What is the relationship of social factors, such as ethnicity and social position, to the level of awareness? Do patients and families with higher levels of education press for more information and are they thus more apt to fall in the category of *open awareness* earlier in their illnesses than people with less education? Does past experience with dying raise the level of awareness of dying people, family members, and other interactors? Are persons in the third and fourth categories more frequently labeled as dying by both health care personnel and lay people than those in the first two categories? Are there other factors yet to be identified which affect the levels of awareness of dying people, their families, and other interactors and which influence interactional behavior?

Allowing for the view that all persons are dying from the moment they are born, there may be a point that can be designated as the beginning of the dying process. This starting point may have both a social and situational definition. The expectations and predictions of health care providers may be important factors in structuring the situation. It is unlikely, however, that the expectations and predictions of health care providers alone explain the wide variations of behaviors among and between those interacting together when someone is perceived as dying. It is more likely that views and expectations of all interactors, including the dying person, are important in structuring the situation of and surrounding the dying person.

The studies discussed identify some of the factors which influence the situation of and surrounding patients and, in turn, the conduct of all involved.

NEED FOR MORE RESEARCH

Despite the proliferation of literature and research about dying and death, some questions which seemed worthwhile for study were left unanswered. These questions became the focus of a research study carried out as a part of the requirements for the Ph.D. degree in Sociology.

Because I am a nurse who continued to practice nursing while completing doctoral study, the hospital environment was open for a participant observation study to examine the variations of behavior of hospitalized dying adults and of persons interacting with them. Focus is upon the interactional and contextual environment where the behavior occurs and which structures interactional patterns and roles.

The purpose of the study is to identify social and interactional factors: patterns, qualities, or processes, that typify the situation of and surrounding the dying person in order to answer the following major questions:

1. Is the *initial* label of dying socially defined? In other words, do people suffer a social death before they are biologically dead?
2. How is a common definition of the situation arrived at when the parameters are unknown, unclear, or taboo? Stated more simply, if the patient's situation is neither known nor understood and is unmentionable, how do all involved come to believe the patient is dying?
3. How are roles created when norms are absent, ill-defined, or conflicting? Stated differently, if no one knows how to act toward a dying person, how are

roles created? More importantly, is there a role for the dying person in contemporary American society that can be described and defined?

REFERENCES

1. Irion PE: The Funeral: Vestige or Value?, New York, Atherton Press, 1966, p. 21
2. Wahl CW: The fear of death. *In* Fulton R (ed): Death and Identity, New York, John Wiley and Sons, Inc., 1965, p. 57
3. Illich I: Medical Nemesis: The Expropriation of Health, New York, Pantheon Books, A Division of Random House, 1976, p. 203
4. Dumong RG, Foss DG: The American View of Death: Acceptance or Denial?, Cambridge, Mass., Schenkman Publishing Co. 1972, p. 2
5. Baker JM, Sorensen KC: A patient's concern with death. Am J Nurs, 63 (July, 1963), 90 — 92; Quint (Benoliel) JC: Nursing services and the care of dying patients: some speculations. Nurs Sci, 2 (Dec., 1964), 432 — 43; Quint (Benoliel) JC, Strauss AL: Nursing students, assignment, and dying patients. Nurs Outlook, 12 (Jan., 1964), 24 — 27; Glaser BG, Strauss AL: Awareness of Dying, Chicago, Aldine Publishing Co., 1965; Mervy F: The plight of dying patients in hospitals. Am J Nurs, 71 (Oct., 1971), 1988 — 90
6. Glaser BG, Strauss AL: Awareness contexts and social interaction. Am Sociol Rev, 29 (Aug.) 669 — 79; Quint (Benoliel) JC: The Nurse and The Dying Patient, New York, Macmillan Company, 1967
7. Kubler-Ross E: On Death and Dying, New York, The Macmillan Company, 1969, p. 10
8. Freud S: Thoughts for the Times on War and Death, London, Hogarth Press, 1957, pp. 275 — 300
9. Kubler-Ross, On Death and Dying, Chap. 1
10. Rosenfeld A: Prolongevity, New York, A Discus Book, published by Avon Books, a division of The Hearst Company, 1976, p. XIX
11. Harrington A: The Immortalist, New York, Random House, 1969
12. Lifton RJ: Survivors of nuclear warfare psychological effects of the atomic bomb in Hiroshima: the theme of death. Daedalus, 92 (1945), 462 — 97; Cohen EA: Human Behavior in the Concentration Camp, New York, W. W. Norton and Co., Inc., 1953; Hoess R: Commandant of Auschwitz, Autobiography, Cleveland, World Publishing Co., 1959 (trs. from German by Constantine Fitzgibbon, 1st ed.); Levi P: Survival in Auschwitz, New York, P. F. Collier Inc., 1961; Hilberg R: The Destruction of the European Jews, Chicago, Ill. Quadrangle Books, 1961
13. Baruch J: Combat death. *In* Schneidman ES (ed): Death: Current Perspectives, Palo Alto, Calif., Mayfield Publishing Company, 1976, p. 94
14. Illich, Medical Nemesis, p. 200
15. Illich, Medical Nemesis, p. 195
16. Illich, Medical Nemesis, p. 195
17. Branson R, Casebeer K, Levine MD, Oden TC, Ramsey P, Capron AM: The Quinlan decision: five commentaries. Institute of Society, Ethics, and the Life Sciences, The Hastings Center Report, 6, no. 1 (Feb. 1976), 8 — 19; Lestz P: A committee to decide quality of life. Am J Nurs, 77, (May, 1977), 862 — 64; McCormick RA: The quality of life, the sanctity of life. Institute of Society, Ethics, and the Life Sciences, the Hastings Center Report, 8, no. 1 (Feb. 1978), 30 — 36
18. Martocchio BC: Death and dying in intensive care units. *In* Daly BJ (ed): Intensive Care Nursing—Current Clinical Nursing Series, Flushing, New York, Medical Examination Publishing Co., Inc., 1980, 441 — 63
19. Curtin L: The Mask of Euthanasia, 2nd ed., Cincinnati, Ohio, N.C.F.L. Inc., 1976; Donovan MI, Pierce SG: Cancer Care Nursing, New York, Appleton-Century-Crofts, A Publishing Division of Prentice-Hall, Inc., 1976, pp. 19 — 33

20. Euthanasia Education Council, 250 W. 57th St., New York 10019, 1978
21. See: Lamerton R: Care of the Dying N. B. The Care and Welfare Library, 1973; Halporn R (ed): The Hospice Concept Essays by Kron, Joan, Robert Buckingham, and Sylvia Lack, et al. and Donna Bates, Brooklyn, New York, Highly Specialized Promotions, 1977; Lack S, Buckingham RW III: First American Hospice: Three Years of Home Care, New Haven, Conn., Dept. of Public Information Hospice, Inc., 1978); Kubler-Ross E, Warshaw M: To Live Until We Say Good-bye, Englewood Cliffs, N.J., Prentice-Hall, Inc., 1978, especially pp. 113 – 149
22. Osis K, Haraldsson E: At the Hour of Death, New York, Avon Books, a Division of Hearst Corporation, 1977; Moody RA Jr.: Life after Life, Atlanta, Mockingbird Books, 1975; Moody RA Jr.; Reflections on Life after Life, Atlanta, Mockingbird Books, 1977
23. Blumer H: Symbolic Interactionism, Perspective and Method, Englewood Cliffs, N.J. Prentice-Hall Inc., 1969
24. Scott CA: Old age and death. Am J Psych, 8 (1896), 67 – 122
25. Lester D: Experimental and correlation studies of fear of death. Psychol Bull, 67 (Jan. 1967, 27 – 36
26. Williams M: Changing attitudes toward death. Human Relations, 19 (Nov., 1966), 405 – 23; Lester D: Experimental and Correlational Studies, 27 – 36
27. Keen S: A day of loving combat, a sketch of Ernest Becker. Psychol Today, 7 (Apr. 1973)
28. Feifel H: Death. In Taboo Topics, 8 – 21
29. Kubler-Ross, On Death and Dying, 1969; Kubler-Ross E: The dying patient's point of view. In Brim O, et al (eds): The Dying Patient, New York, The Russell Sage Foundation, 1970, pp. 156 – 172
30. Glaser and Strauss, Awareness of Dying, 1965
31. Kalish RA: The onset of the dying process. Omega, 1 (1970), 57 – 69
32. Kubler-Ross, On Death and Dying, p. 262
33. Kubler-Ross, On Death and Dying
34. Weisman AD: The Realization of Death: A Guide for the Psychological Autopsy, New York, J. Aronson, 1974
35. Schultz R, Aderman D: Clinical research and the stages of dying. Omega, 7 (1974), 137 – 143
36. Shibles W: Death: An Interdisciplinary Analysis, Whitewater, Wisc., Language Press, 1974
37. Pattison EM: The Experience of Dying, Englewood Cliffs, N.J., Prentice-Hall, 1977, p. 306
38. Glaser and Strauss, Awareness Contexts and Social Interaction, p. 669; Glaser and Strauss, Awareness of Dying
39. Kutscher AH (ed): Death and Bereavement, Springfield, Ill. Charles Thomas, 1969; Schoenberg B, Carr AC, Peretz D, Kutscher AH (eds): Loss and Grief: Psychological Management in Medical Practice, New York, Columbia University Press, 1970 and Psychosocial Aspects of Terminal Care, New York, Columbia University Press, 1972; Pincus L: Death and the Family: The Importance of Mourning, New York, Random House, Vintage Books, 1974; Schiff HS: The Bereaved Parent, New York, Crown Publishers, Inc., 1977
40. Alsop S: Stay of Execution, New York, J. B. Lippincott Company, 1973; Lund D: Eric, New York, J. B. Lippincott Company, 1974; Lazarus W: The thing in Harry Sapir's side. Cleveland (Magazine), 3 (Sept., 1974), 53 – 60; Hendin D: Death as a Fact of Life, New York, Warner Publication Paperback Edition, 1974
41. Glaser B, Strauss A: Status Passage, Chicago, Aldine Atherton, 1971
42. Glaser B, Strauss A: Temporal Aspects of Dying as a Nonscheduled Status Passage, Chicago, Aldine Publishing Company, 1970

3   Theoretical and Sensitizing Concepts

SOCIAL INTERACTION AND BEHAVIOR

The purpose of the study, as described at the end of Chapter 2, I felt could be achieved by observing the behavior of hospitalized dying adults and by examining the differences in behavior in terms of the interactional and contextual environment in which they occurred. I also believed that such information would contribute to better understanding and greater acceptance of these differences.

There was no reason to believe that the behavior of dying people comes about in any different way than the behavior of those interacting with them. Thus, I assumed that the behavior of dying people, just as the behavior of those interacting with them is developed through social interaction.

When human beings interact with one another, they take into account what each other is doing or about to do; they then direct their own behavior in terms of what they have taken into account. Thus, the activities of others are factors in the formation of any person's behavior. In the face of actions of others, a person may abandon an intention or purpose, revise it, check or suspend it, intensify it or replace it (1). In addition to the above, I would add that people interact within an environment that may diminish or enhance interacting with each other and thus influence behavior.

Focusing upon interactional behavior and environmental conditions does not negate the impact of physiological changes upon behavior. It emphasizes that how individuals perceive and react to physiological changes are equally important; however, it is not the physiological condition, per se, that elicits the behavior. It is the interpretation or meaning of the condition in conjunction with social interaction and the context of the situation that elicits behavior. Therefore, in order to understand behavior, it is important to discover each observed person's interpretation of the condition.

Although no attempt was made to form a series of premature conceptualizations to fix and bind the phenomenon of dying behavior, some sociological theories and concepts were used to generate pertinent questions or to offer some possible explanations for behavioral differences. Some of these concepts, in turn, constituted variables for observations. The specification of the concepts as variables did not preclude the observation of other factors or the identification and use of other theories and concepts that arose in the empirical setting and were helpful to the study. Socialization is the first concept discussed.

SOCIALIZATION

Literature on socialization emphasizes early socialization and less often socialization throughout the life cycle (2), but clearly stops short of socialization or resocialization into a role which is consonant with termination of life or termination of other relationships.

Socialization refers to "the process by which individuals acquire knowledge, skills, and dispositions that enable them to participate as more or less effective members of groups and society (3)." Since it is difficult to discuss socialization without introducing the concept of role, a social role is defined as the behaviors expected of an individual occupying a given social position (4).

Social learning occurs throughout the life cycle and within each of the various groups and organizational contexts that provide settings for social behavior. Human behavior does not occur in social isolation. Even the acts an individual performs when alone are to a great extent influenced by significant others in the individual's life span.

Socialization is a two-way process. Both the socializing agent and the novice are learners; the emphasis is one of degree. The learner consciously makes choices, seeks out behaviors which are acceptable, and decides, as well as is induced, to acquire new skills or to alter existing behavior within various contexts.

Socialization also involves both deliberate and incidental learning on the part of the individual being socialized and on the part of the socializers. Social learning occurs in a social environment and the learners are an integral part of that environment. The learners respond to stimuli from others around them and at the same time their responses constitute stimuli for those responsible for socializing them. The learners then, to a variable extent, help to shape their own environment and become socializers as well as learners.

In the face of unclear norms and vaguely defined role expectations, it is difficult to know who is the socializer and who the learner, as is the case in interactions between dying people and others. Although many authors write in terms of the socializer and the learner, it may be a purely analytical distinction. In the dying-interactor situation, there may be an alternating sequence with the interactors changing from one role to the other.

When it comes to dying, it not only is difficult to identify who is the socializer and who is the learner; it is also difficult to identify what is being learned, and how the information is transmitted. The problem is not so much that society completely fails to socialize its members in regard to dying, but that society fails to socialize its members in a fashion that is consonant with the chronicity of dying and the interactions with others during this period of living-while-knowingly-dying.

Socializing people to believe that dying and death are taboo topics or not addressing death at all is as much a form of teaching as is addressing the subject openly. Because society fails to socialize individuals in some deliberate fashion does not preclude incidental processes of learning which serve an anticipatory function. For instance, religious doctrines may contribute to learning varying responses to dying. Views of the meaning of death and dying may also be influenced by social position, ethnic origin, and even occupation. Past experiences with dying persons, or stories about dying persons, may also contribute to learning. How much or what kinds of incidental learning regarding dying occurs in everyday interactions remains open to question.

Interactors enter the situation not only with differentially developed skills and competencies resulting from prior socialization, but with different perceptions from which to appraise the situation. These differences in skills, competencies, and perceptions may provide or promote different options for behavior and offer some explanation for the variations in interactional patterns.

TERMINATING RELATIONSHIPS

How does American society prepare its members for dying? Or perhaps a more pertinent question, does American society prepare its members for dying or for ending relationships?

It is as important for society to socialize people for ending relationships as it is for establishing them. Living is marked by a series of terminations of relationships. Moving from one location to another, graduations from various schools, promotions, and retirement are some examples of situations in which relationships may be permanently severed. There is the possibility that relationships will be maintained and that promises to keep in touch, write, or telephone will be kept, but there are no guarantees. Death removes any doubt. Relationships will be ended. Problems arise for the dying person and the interactors when dying is perceived as synonymous with death.

Dying has become a chronic process with the end point, death, perceived as inevitable. But dying is also a part of living. To maintain quality of living during the period of living-while-knowingly-dying, it is imperative to socialize people for terminating relationships. If people gained competence in dealing with terminating relationships throughout their lives, they should be better able to maintain interactional relationships preceding death. If there is to be quality of living during this living-while-knowingly-dying period, the continuation or discontinuation of interactional relationships should be based upon mutual decision. It should not be due to a lack of competence in interacting in the situation, nor to poorly defined role expectations.

ROLE AND ROLE FORMATION

The variations in the behavior of people when facing imminent death may reflect the poorly defined status of this role. Is there a dying role? Are there identifiable role expectations for dying persons and those with whom they interact regarding the role of each, and each other's view of the other?

There are several definitions of role. To theorists like Parsons (5), Merton, (6), Gross et al. (7), Biddle and Thomas (8), every social position has a role and status attached to it. A *role* is a set of expectations legitimately expected of the occupant and status is the behavior the occupant is legitimately entitled to expect of specified others. *Role performance* consists of conforming behaviorally to these expectations. This definition implies a relatively predetermined, stable set of mutual expectations. No attention is paid to what occurs in situations where status is not accorded. It is a view of roles and relationships as a part of a pre-existing framework which is then imposed upon the interactors. This view of roles focuses upon the functions and basic needs of society, with people behaving in certain ways to maintain society by fulfilling basic societal needs and functions.

McCall and Simmons (9) state that this is a limited model observed only in unusual circumstances, as in tightly structured organizations in which roles are formally defined. In actuality, even in highly structured organizations, such as hospitals, there is a continuum ranging from highly structured to relatively non-structured roles. Regardless of the degree of structure, there are still variations in how any individual acts out his role. However, these variations are somewhat determined by the general mutual expectations and goals of the defined role which existed prior to the individuals entering the situation and as such provides some structure. Nonetheless, the questions of how roles develop and how the system remains stable are pertinent.

Goslin (10) suggests that the stability of the interactional system depends upon agreement among participants as to what each may expect of the other, a view that is consistent with that of the *symbolic interactionists*. Symbolic inter-actionists stress linguistic and gestural communications, especially the role of language in the formation of the mind, the self, and the society. They (11) propose that the self is created in interaction with others specifically through language and the ability to take the role of others. They maintain that people behave as they do because of their perceptions of what they ought to do and how others will react to their behavior. Symbolic interactionists' emphasis upon the negotiation of meaning and behavior in individual and group encounters, and the perspec-tives of various actors in defining the situation in some fashion common to all, is of particular importance. Their general focus is on the *needs* and *behavior* of people as *individuals* rather than the *aggregate needs* of *society*. Social roles de-velop as similar interactions are repeatedly agreed upon. The symbolic interac-tionists, then, explain interpersonal behavior and the development of social roles. They do not account for the existence of and persistence of social structures, which is of major concern to the *structural functionalists*.

Although the interactionist and structural functionalist views are not entirely compatible in the assumptions they make about mankind, they are not mutually exclusive when looking at roles. Their difference may be in emphasis upon process or structure. Each view is useful in explaining a particular aspect of the total picture. In addition, each view either implicitly or explicitly alludes to the need for agreement among and between interactors about the situation and what is occurring—or, stated differently, the need for the development of a com-mon definition of the situation by the interactors and their negotiation for mutu-ally acceptable roles.

In any interactional system, each participant influences the behavior of each of the other participants. Agreement arises through a process of bargaining or negotiating in which all participants alter their behavior until there is consensus as to what each may expect of the other (12). Consensus is defined as the lack of impeding disagreements, not agreement on all appraisals among all interactors (13). Thus consensus can develop whether or not there is a pre-existing formal-ized role structure.

Berger and Luckman (14) attend both to the individual actors and to social institutions by distinguishing between subjective and objective reality. *Objective reality* exists beyond the person. *Subjective reality* is that which is internalized by the person. It is what is meaningful to him or her. It is an individual identity transmitted through socialization. A social role then has an objective reality that existed before the person occupied it or even perceived it. Yet, a social role must be subjectively real to the person who occupies it. Basically, Berger and Luckman describe a dialectic relationship. Society is a human product, created by human acts and interactors, and the person is a social product. Each individual's identity is subjectively real, yet is determined by such objective social facts as social class and other demographic factors, as well as interaction with others.

Social institutions and roles arise in interactions which become habitual. They become institutionalized as future generations are socialized to them. Consequently, although reality is socially created, it is perceived as objectively real. The notion that perceived reality is always in the process of construction by the interactors in addition to being a pre-existing phenomenon is especially important when studying dying person-interactor relationships.

In dying person-interactor relationships there may be institutionalized norms or role prescriptions. If indeed, there are relatively few norms or role prescriptions, then satisfactory patterns of role accommodation must be achieved primarily through the process of role negotiation. In other words, mutually acceptable reciprocal roles must be developed for both dying persons and those interacting with them. The role of dying persons, as well as those interacting with them, then, is constantly unfolding and evolving. Roles are negotiated in interactions with significant others and are always in the process of shifting.

NEGOTIATIONS FOR ROLE AND SOCIAL IDENTITY

Negotiation is the process of bargaining over the terms of social rewards and their contingent gratifications which may be extrinsic (material goods, information), or intrinsic (role support, bodily pleasures), or mixed (15). In discussing the dynamics of interactions, McCall and Simmons (16) describe two stages in bargaining: the negotiation of social identity and the negotiation of interactive roles. They suggest that agreement must first be reached on who each person is to the others in terms of social categories, for example, physician, nurse, patient, visitor, before bargaining can begin on the specific content of the present behavior of the actors. Agreement on social category and content is motivated by cost reward considerations.

Each person seeks to incorporate into one's performance in the situation a role that takes into account other persons and the relative importance of the parts the other persons play. If this understanding is not in gross conflict with what other persons understand their roles to be, a working agreement is said to have been reached. The interactors then continue to negotiate for their specific interactive roles, based upon this working agreement which defines the situation.

The question of whether this negotiation is a person-to-person process which goes on in each situation is important to consider since health care providers would be repeating the process time and time again under similar conditions, whereas dying patients and others might not be repeating the process. It is possible that experience in negotiating for roles offers greater options for behavior.

For McCall and Simmons (17), the definition of the situation is the beginning of the process of negotiating for role and social identity. It is subject to change as factors in the interaction change. It persists only as long as there is correspondence of the constituent processes. If anyone behaves in an unexpected fashion, the process begins again; a new agreement is negotiated. Further, a single encounter may present the appearance of successive phases of interaction, each marked by the negotiation of a new working agreement.

McCall and Simmons take exception to the view of Goffman (18), who suggests that in any encounter attention is focused upon the matters involved in a particular situation. Boundaries are set by *transformation rules* (19) which govern what is allowed to intrude upon that encounter. Identities of participants and transformation rules make up the definition of the situation. When matters that have been declared irrelevant or unreal by the transformation rules intrude, tension results. For Goffman, "The coherence and persistence of a focused gathering depends upon maintaining a boundary, so the integrity of this barrier seems to depend upon the management of tensions." Efforts of the interactors then are directed towards dealing with the tension which represents a threat to the entire encounter. Conversely, it would seem that dealing with tension could serve as a means for holding a gathering together by giving it a common focus.

Nonetheless, in any negotiation process some parties bargain from positions of greater strength. In this regard, it is conceivable that those who most accurately assess the negotiability of role expectations have significant advantage over other participants (20). Thus when nurses and physicians are patients, they would be expected to make more demands for information than lay persons. Scheff's (21) study of psychiatric and legal interviews supports this view since it demonstrated that interactors who recognized the bargaining aspects of the transaction had greater power in defining the entire situation.

The distribution of power in the relationship is another aspect of interactional systems. The effect of power in role relationships is difficult to assess. In terms of dying people, it would appear that the physician, in particular, and other health professionals, in general, possess a great deal of legitimate power and thus may be in a better negotiating position than is the patient. On the other hand, the obligations which accompany this power may limit the freedom professionals have in negotiating for roles. For instance, the nurse may feel obligated to follow the physician's edicts although she may disagree. Consequently, individuals in designated subordinate roles, which do not carry the same obligations, including the patient, significant others, and semi-professional workers, may be in a better bargaining position. Of importance is the point that when negotiation occurs, it occurs within the structural constraints imposed by the formal role. Another crucial factor regarding power and thus role negotiations is the control of resources, including information. Regardless of the formal and informal distribution of authority or power, the member who possesses such resources has considerable power. While possession of information grants power, it may also serve to inhibit freedom of interaction when, for example, the knowledge is threatening to a relationship.

Another factor to be considered is the internalization of values and standards of conduct which may restrict one's freedom to negotiate. This may be especially true in interactions concerning the dying person, where institutional prescriptions are unclear and, consequently, relationships may be based on personal power.

As a result of the taboo nature of the topic of dying, individuals may find themselves committed to playing their roles in specific ways as a consequence of having played them that way before. The evasive behavior of health professionals in regard to interacting with the dying is an example of such role playing. Behavior may have evolved from not knowing what else to do for so long that it became a habit. Habitual or ritualistic behavior may lead to relinquishing the options for negotiating for mutually acceptable roles.

Many questions related to dying persons remain unanswered. What occurs in the situation of dying persons where there may not be a consensus about the situation and perhaps little structure arising from normatively defined roles and statuses? In this situation does negotiation occur? How do dying persons become free to negotiate in a situation where they may not recognize the possibility for negotiating? If they do recognize the possibility for negotiating, are they given the opportunity to do so? How do dying individuals exercise their right to expect certain behavior of others in the interactional system, when they may know neither their rights nor what to expect? The same question may be raised with reference to all persons who interact with dying persons.

The variations of behavior observed among dying patients may be attributed in part to the fact that the roles themselves become subject to the idiosyncrasies of discrete negotiations. The question remains, however, what additional factors or variables contribute to variations in behavior? Indiscriminant application of concepts or labels such as denial is one such factor.

DENIAL, AN INTERPERSONAL PHENOMENON

In the absence of institutionalized norms, sanctions, role prescriptions, or structure of some kind, the interactions following the discovery that death is imminent may take precedence over previous interactional experiences in influencing behavior. In such highly unstructured situations the participants may reach out to many other interactors. The other interactors may respond to the dying person in a noncommital or ambiguous way, may avoid responding at all, or may avoid the dying person. The ambiguity of the response, as well as the structure of the situation and probable knowledge of death as a taboo subject, may lead to the dying person's withdrawal from the situation. This withdrawal from the situation may represent avoidance behavior; however, it is avoidance generated by either the ambiguity or the covert structure of the situation and is in response to the ambiguous non-interpretable behaviors of the other interactors.

Some individuals would interpret this avoidance or withdrawal behavior (whether on the part of the dying or interactor) solely as a function of the intrapsychic defense mechanism called *denial*. Anna Freud (22) suggests that denial as a response to danger is basic to other defense mechanisms. It is the most primitive defense serving as a unifying concept for different defenses. She did not suggest, however, that denial is a unitary mechanism which serves to repudiate reality. Unfortunately, the concept of denial has been expanded and has come to be generally defined as the kind of observed behavior that suggests a failure to accept an obvious fact or its significance to the individual involved in the situation. Denial is not only presented as a well-defined entity which is assumed to arise out of some inner or intrapsychic mechanism; it is also viewed as a static phenomenon which can be used as an explanatory concept. When this occurs,

43

the term becomes synonymous with the facts. As a result, there is at least tacit discouragement of further inquiry into the reason for withdrawal behaviors which may contribute to limiting interaction (23).

For example, based upon my clinical observations, it is not unusual to hear people say, "he is using denial," or "she is denying her illness." These inferences seem to reflect the expectation that people facing their own or another's death will be upset, at least initially; if the person remains calm, the behavior is attributed to denial. The behaviors of staff members are explained in a similar fashion. For instance, whether a staff member avoids interacting with a dying patient or seems too comfortable in interacting with a dying person, the behavior is often labeled as denial by peers. Observers seem to explain behaviors that are different from their expectations by concluding that denial is operant. Use of denial in these situations suggests that the sole purpose of denial is to mitigate the meaning of some external danger. It implies that it is some intrapsychic mechanism that arises in response to acute anxiety.

However, apparent avoidance behaviors may not be simply manifestations of intrapsychic processes. Rather, avoidance behaviors may be contingent upon how interactors interpret what each other is doing or about to do, and then direct their own behaviors accordingly. Is it possible, then, that denial may be viewed as a process which emerges out of certain styles of interaction? If so, the concept of denial is itself an interpersonal, not intrapsychic, phenomenon. It is not an established intrapsychic phenomenon which is available when a person is threatened. It is a label applied by an observer when the behaviors of the observed do not "fit" the expectations which arise from his or her own definition of the situation. It may or may not be consonant with how the observed defines the situation.

Thus the application of the term may become a convenient label or stereotype. As such it may preclude further inquiry into a situation and contribute to limiting further interactions. For instance, if a patient's non-compliance to treatment is attributed to denial of the illness, there is no incentive to search for other explanations of the non-compliant behavior. In fact, there is no reason to continue the interaction, at least as it relates to the non-compliant behavior. The results of limiting interactions are decreased opportunities for roles which might lead to a more stable relationship and for developing a common definition of the situation by health care providers and the dying person that would be more acceptable to both. In this case, W. I. Thomas's dictum, "if men define situations as real, they are real in their consequences" fits the situation.

However, the application of such labels as *denial* or its counterpart, *acceptance*, by interactors may also represent an attempt on the part of the labelers to structure the situation by imposing a definition on it. The definition may provide a baseline for developing informal norms to govern interactive behavior. Thus, stereotyping of behavior may be functional for the labeler since it provides structure to an ambiguous situation, but dysfunctional to the dying person-interactor relationship, especially if a particular kind of interaction is presumed to be *good*.

A label then can be a variable which influences interaction. Of equal importance is the use of the labeling perspective as a process, especially in regard to the questions "when, by whom, and under what circumstances is the hospitalized person defined as dying?"

LABELING

It is possible that the *initial* label of dying is at least in part socially defined. Dying can be seen as an *ascribed status* which reflects not only the physiological or pathological changes of the person but the responses of other people as well (24). In addition, people may initiate the label themselves.

The introduction of the notion of labeling at first seems paradoxical to the view that all actors are significant in shaping their own behavior according to their interpretations of the interactional situation. However, if one conceptualizes labeling in the same fashion as role negotiating, it is not so paradoxical, since both processes enable interactors to define their situation. Labeling, as does role negotiating, occurs within an organizational setting with varying power relationships (25).

As alluded to in the discussion of denial, labeling or stereotyping may have considerable impact upon behavior and interactions. Studies of mental illness (26) suggest that stereotyped images of mental illness are, to some extent, learned in early childhood and that these stereotypes are inadvertently reaffirmed in ordinary social interaction. One researcher (27) believes that traditional stereotypes of mental illness are not discarded, even by those who are familiar with psychiatric concepts, and continue to exist alongside the medical conceptions. These stereotypes are maintained because they receive almost continual support from the mass media and in social discourse.

Although no empirical data exist at present, it is conceivable there are such stereotypes regarding dying. The fact that the subject of dying is taboo and that dying persons frequently die in hospitals, nursing homes, and other institutions in which they are segregated from other members of society, suggest a negative stereotype. Walter Lippman's (28) classic description of the "pictures in our minds" which color everyday interactions, is pertinent when analyzing reactions to dying individuals. As he stated, "we do not first see then define, we define first and then see."

The dying label may carry with it certain rights and privileges not accorded to those who are not considered to be dying. On the other hand, it may also act as a constraint on the behavior of people so labeled, thus limiting the possibilities for negotiating for roles that are more acceptable to them.

SUMMARY

The behavior of dying people, and of those interacting with them, is developed through social interaction. The nature of the interaction is influenced by the contextual environment and by factors within the interactional environment. To understand the differences in the behavior of dying people and of those interacting with them, it is necessary to explore the social processes that underlie and, in turn, influence these behaviors.

Further, it is postulated that observation of dying persons without exploration and understanding of the underlying social process negates the development of greater competencies in caring for the dying, and limits options for changing the behavior of health care providers, dying persons, or those interacting with them.

45

Practical concerns, combined with clinical experiences with dying persons and review of the literature, led to the following research purpose and associated questions. In this study, no attempt was made to answer all the questions, although they were all important and worthy of exploration. Instead, they were used as sensitizing questions that provided guides for making observations.

PURPOSE OF STUDY AND SENSITIZING QUESTIONS

The purpose of the study was to identify patterns, processes, or qualities which typify the situation of and surrounding dying persons. The following questions were explored.

1. Is the INITIAL label of dying socially defined and differentially applied?
    a. Under what conditions is a person initially defined as dying (e.g., what is the relationship of social factors such as social class, occupation, religion, and past experience with other dying people to the timing of the initial label)?
    b. What is the process through which the label evolves?
    c. With whom does the label originate and how is it legitimized?
    d. What happens if an incorrect label is applied?
2. How is a common definition of the situation arrived at when the parameters are either unknown or taboo?
    a. Is there an *implicit,* common definition of the situation? If so, under what circumstances does it arise and how does it affect interaction? How is it recognized?
    b. Is there an *explicit,* common definition of the situation? If so, under what conditions does it arise, and how does it affect the interactions? How is it recognized?
    c. Are there identifiable patterns of communication which contribute to or detract from arriving at a common definition of the situation?
    d. Do social factors, such as socioeconomic class, religious background, and previous socialization, influence the process of arriving at some consensus or a common definition of the situation?
    e. If a common definition of the situation is arrived at, are others inducted into it? If so, how?
    f. What are the consequences of arriving at a common definition which is false?
3. How are interactive roles formed under conditions of relative normlessness, or where norms are either unknown or ill-defined or conflicting?
    a. Are there commonly accepted rules and sanctions for behavior for all interactors which can be identified?
    b. Are there commonalities among interactors in an expected role for the dying person? If so, how structured or ambiguous is it? How do various expectations conflict?
    c. Is there anticipatory socialization, however poorly defined and implicit, for dying? If so, what form does it take?
    d. Do social factors, such as socioeconomic class, educational background, and prior experience, influence the process of role formation or the type of role formed?

e. Assuming that there is negotiation for role, what are the patterns of negotiation?

    i. What factors influence negotiations (e.g., power, information, social factors)?

    ii. If the individual is less able to verbalize one's role effectively, is that role more likely to be defined by others, and will social constraints determine behavior?

f. Will role negotiations occur through an intermediary acting on behalf of the family, dying person, or health professionals? If so, who acts as an intermediary for whom, and under what circumstances?

g. Do patterns of role negotiations and expectations of roles of all interactors differ as a person is perceived to be closer to death?

    i. Will there be greater or lesser constraints on each interactor's behavior? If so, what forms will they take?

    ii. Will all roles become more or less structural, or more or less ritualized?

REFERENCES

1. Blumer H: Symbolic Interactionism, Perspective and Method, Englewood Cliffs, N.J., Prentice-Hall, Inc., 1969
2. Brim O, Jr.: Socialization through the life cycle. In Orville Brim, Jr. and S. Wheeler (eds): Socialization After Childhood, New York, Wiley, 1966
3. Brim, Socialization, 1966
4. Gross NC, Mason WS, McAcheen AW: Explorations in Role Analysis: Studies in School Superintendency Role, New York, Wiley, 1958
5. Parsons T: The Social System, New York, Free Press, 1951
6. Merton RK: Social Theory and Social Structure, (revised ed.), Glencoe, Ill., Free Press of Glencoe, 1957, especially Chapter 9
7. Gross, Mason, McAcheen, Explorations in Role Analysis, 1958
8. Biddle BJ, Thomas EJ: Role Theory: Concepts and Research, New York, Wiley, 1966
9. McCall GJ, Simmons JL: Identities and Interactions: An Examination of Human Associations in Everyday Life, New York, Free Press, 1966
10. Goslin D: Introduction. In Handbook of Socialization Theory and Research, Chicago, Rand McNally and Company, 1969, p. 7
11. Mead GH: Mind, Self and Society, Chicago, University of Chicago Press, 1934; Cooley CH: Human Nature and the Social Order, New York, Schocken Books, 1964; Cottrell L: Interpersonal interaction and the development of self. In Goslin D (ed): Handbook of Socialization Theory and Research, Chicago, Rand McNally and Company, 1969, pp. 543 – 70
12. Mead, Mind, Self, Society
13. McCall and Simmons, Identities and Interactions, p. 127
14. Berger PL, Luckman T: The Social Construction of Reality, Garden City, N.J., Anchor Books, Doubleday, 1967
15. See, for example: Brown JS: The Motivation of Behavior, New York, McGraw-Hill, 1961; Blau P: Exchange and Power in Social Life, New York, Wiley, 1964
16. McCall and Simmons, Identities and Interactions, pp. 140 – 66
17. McCall and Simmons, Identities and Interactions
18. Goffman I: Encounters: Two Studies in the Sociology of Interactions, Indianapolis, Bobbs Merrill Company, 1961, pp. 7 – 81
19. Goffman, Encounters, p. 33

20. See, for example: Goslin, Socialization Theory and Research, pp. 8 – 10
21. Scheff T: Negotiating reality: notes on power in the assessment of responsibility. Social Problems, 16 (1968), 3 – 17
22. Freud A: The Ego and Mechanisms of Defense, trans. C. Bains, London: Hogarth Press, Ltd., and The Institute of Psychoanalysis, 1948
23. Weisman A: On Death and Denying, New York, Behavioral Publications, Inc., 1972, pp. 52 – 64
24. Erickson K: Notes on the sociology of deviance. Social Problems, 9 (Spring), 308
25. Shur EM: Labeling Deviant Behavior, New York, Harper and Row, 1971, p. 8
26. Scheff T: Being Mentally Ill, Chicago, Aldine Publishing Co. 1966
27. Nunnally JC: Popular Conceptions of Mental Health, New York, Holt-Rinehart-Winston, 1961
28. Lippman W: Public Opinions, New York, The MacMillan Company, 1922

4   The Research Strategy

PARTICIPANT OBSERVATION

P articipant observation was selected as the most appropriate method for collecting data for this study. Participant observation, a research method commonly used in sociology and anthropology, makes use of various data collecting techniques. These include: observation, interviewing, review of available documents, and participation with self analysis. Participant observation is an unstructured approach in which the researcher participates in and observes face-to-face interactions in the natural setting. Observations are guided, described, and then analyzed in terms of the investigator's theoretical perspectives (1).

Participant observation emphasizes the importance of making on-going evaluation so that the researcher may change the research focus at any stage of inquiry while still maintaining sight of the major research objectives. This method was selected to investigate the complex questions regarding dying because it allowed me to maintain flexibility in observations, methods of data collection, sources of data, methods of analysis and interpretation. Flexibility across these stages of inquiry was desired because it promoted continual interplay among the research setting, research methods, and known and emerging theory.

As a sociologist and a registered nurse with a Master's degree in nursing, I was employed as a part-time staff nurse prior to designing the study. The feasibility of conducting a participant observation study in the natural setting was evaluated during the period of employment. Several factors were considered before deciding that the research could realistically be conducted in the *natural* setting. These factors were: (1) the nature of the patient population; (2) my ability to establish effective working relationships with other staff members; (3) my acceptance as a competent nurse by the patients, nursing staff, and physicians; (4) the accessibility of observations and information pertinent to the objectives of this study without manipulation or introduction of major changes in the environment; (5) the feasibility of adhering to the policies and accepted practices of the institution while collecting pertinent data; and (6) the acceptance of patients and their families of informal discussions concerning their illnesses.

COLLECTING THE DATA

Data were collected over a two-year period. During this time I spent an average of 20 hours per week on selected patient care units. Data were collected at all hours during the day or night with most being collected during the day shift, 7:00 a.m. to 4:00 p.m., or during the evening shift, 4:00 p.m. to midnight. Additional time was spent within the medical center in: (1) informal interactions with hospital personnel, patients, and families; (2) reviewing medical records; and (3) attending other professional and social gatherings in which data pertinent to the objectives of this study were available.

SETTING AND INTERACTIONAL ENVIRONMENT

The study was conducted in a large midwestern medical center which was oriented toward cure or at least toward the maintenance of optimum functioning for each individual. Two adult care units purposely were selected for this study. One was a 36-bed medical unit, the other a surgical intensive care unit. Most of the data were collected on the 36-bed patient care unit, which housed private service medical patients. These patients, men and women over 13 years old, had physical pathology which was being treated medically. Approximately one-third had fatal illnesses.

The patients were under the immediate care of their private physicians; however, a resident physician and three interns were assigned to the unit to implement and coordinate the medical care of these patients. A different resident was assigned to the unit monthly. Each intern was assigned for a three-month rotation; starting dates varied. Each intern was assigned selected patients and followed them throughout his or her rotation. Patients, although assigned to one intern, at times had more than one intern involved in their care on any one admission, and many interns over several admissions.

An important factor in selecting this unit, in addition to the nature of the patient population, was that nursing personnel were permanently scheduled to work there, and generally were assigned to the same patients each day they worked. These factors offered some continuity of interactions.

Although this unit serviced private patients, the third party payment system facilitated delivery of care to a cross section of socioeconomic classes. Because there were few indigent patients on the unit, direct observation of the lowest socioeconomic class was not possible. Data regarding staff service patients were obtained from physicians and nurses who worked there.

The second division selected was a surgical intensive care unit (SICU), with a 13-bed capacity. This was a large rectangular room with beds placed in a "U" shape along three walls. Both private and staff patients were cared for on this unit. It was equipped with the latest in lifesaving equipment and staffed by highly skilled personnel who were permanently assigned to this division. The SICU was designed to assist patients through acute life-threatening situations. As such, it offered a contrast to the social and environmental milieu of the 36-bed medical unit. Consequently, it served both as a source for exploring variations in structural effects, role relationships, and the definitions of the *dying patient* and as a means for determining generalizability of findings. Neither admission to the medical center nor assignment to either unit defined the situation or inadvertently labeled the patient as dying.

SAMPLE

The sample comprised 47 patients between the ages of 14 and 88 years, to whom I gave nursing care and who met any or all of the following criteria: (1) they were believed to have a limited life span by virtue of their diagnostic label or guarded prognosis; (2) they had observable physical deterioration or non-remitting progressive symptoms; (3) the patient or family defined that death was imminent, regardless of medical opinion.

PROCEDURE FOR SAMPLE SELECTION

As a staff nurse, I was assigned to care for patients as dictated by the needs of the unit(s) or the severity of illness of the patients. At times my assignments were made by other registered nurses functioning as team leaders. At other times, I served as nursing team leader and selected my own patients, in addition to being responsible for the 12 to 18 patients which constituted a team load. In the latter instance, the assignment to a team was made by another registered nurse. Even as a team leader, the patients I cared for were dictated by the particular structure of the team in terms of (1) capabilities of available workers also assigned to the team, and (2) the acuity of illness and the complexity of care required by patients for whom the assigned personnel were responsible. Consequently, I necessarily cared for some patients who were not subjects in this study. Patients fitting the criteria for the sample assigned to me became subjects and were followed throughout their hospital stay and on subsequent hospitalizations. It is common practice for nurses to freely interact with all patients whether or not they are assigned to care for them. Thus, following patients to whom one was not assigned was customary and did not change the natural flow of events.

In this study there was no attempt to control for the length of hospital stay, diagnosis, or attending physician, although these data were recorded. It was not expected that the patients in the sample would necessarily die in the hospital. The focus was on the dialogue between these seriously ill patients and those interacting with them and not the actual event of death.

HOW THE DATA WERE COLLECTED

Because participant observation in the natural setting was used, there were no formal interviews. Data were collected during normal interactions with subjects. Other interactions related to the study were also recorded.

As a staff nurse, I assumed the responsibilities, obligations, and privileges customary to that role. This included access to multiple sources of data relevant to the objectives of this study. In addition to the interactions with dying patients, their families, and significant others and health care practitioners, there was open access to meetings and conferences, physicians' rounds, and informal and formal discussions related to dying persons and those interacting with them.

Participant Observation. Three variations of participant observation were used in collecting data. First, I participated as an observer. At these times, I was physically present, but refrained from active verbal or nonverbal participation. For instance, I would observe interactions and listen to conversations between patients and others, and between health care practitioners. I also attended conferences and reports but did not actively participate in them.

Second, in informal gatherings such as coffee breaks, lunch breaks, or other social gatherings not held in the immediate patient care areas, I participated, but as a researcher. In these instances, I intentionally looked for opportunities to direct the conversation toward topics related to the study. Sharing of hospital experiences during such informal gatherings is common among nurses and other health care providers, consequently, it is not difficult nor inappropriate to obtain data in these situations.

The third variation was to maintain a dual role, that of actively participating as both nurse and as researcher. With this approach I freely participated in the workings of the patient care division, contributed to discussions, and administered nursing care to patients. When using this approach, I was consciously making observations, taking notes, and was mindful that observed events, including my own participation, would be recorded later.

Field Notes Made in the Hospital. Following each observational period, all interactions, observations, and conversations were tape-recorded in diary form. Where appropriate, field notes were written during or shortly following the actual observed event. In most instances, it was possible to jot down rough notes since nurses customarily write notes to use as guides in writing nursing notes, care plans, and in giving reports on their assigned patients. In instances where note taking was not possible or where it was inappropriate, I relied on recall to reconstruct interactions and observations. In all instances, field notes were taperecorded within eight hours of the observation period.

Because a professional typist transcribed the tapes, two precautions were taken: (1) all subjects and their interactors were identified by case number or initials prior to taping to assure anonymity; and (2) all transcriptions were verified by simultaneously listening to the tape and reading the transcriptions before the tapes were erased or the original rough notes were discarded. Much credit is to be given to the typist. No tapes were lost; and the transcriptions were perfect with the exception of minor spelling errors and occasional changes in wording which were easily corrected. The transcriptions constituted the data for analysis.

In addition to the notes made about interactions, other sources of data were used. These sources are described next.

Medical Records. After receiving permission, present and past medical records were reviewed on each subject. Data about the family structure and history, as well as all hospitalizations related to the present illnesses, were recorded. Such factors as length of stay, course of illness and treatment, and functional ability of the patient during each hospitalization were included. In addition, data related to the objectives were compiled from physicians' progress notes and nurses' notes.

Nursing Care Plans. The plans developed by nurses for a patient's care were another source of data. The nursing care plans include a succinct summary of the patient's past medical history and present illness; the patient's perception of the illness as perceived by the nurse; the patient's eating and sleeping patterns; usual life-style, including occupation; and a statement of goals for the patient's care, including interventions nursing personnel must take to achieve the stated goals (see Appendix).

Informants. Health care providers, patients, and visitors became informants for the study. Through the course of normal conversations, they kept me up to date on the whereabouts of the patients who had left the hospital, and shared their observations about patients. They also answered questions regarding the meaning of certain language and suggested ways to gain access to additional information. Nurses and others told me about films, conferences, and workshops which they felt were related to the study.

THE PROBLEMS OF PARTICIPANT OBSERVATION

ENTRY INTO THE SITUATION

Because of the sensitive topic and subject matter of this study, I anticipated problems in gaining permission to conduct the study. In reality there were fewer problems than anticipated. The proposal was submitted to the appropriate research review committees and approved with minimal difficulty. Some physician members of one review committee personally interviewed me. They raised questions as to whether data could be obtained without upsetting patients and their families. Researchers unfamiliar with the method of participation observation expressed concern over whether "appropriate data" could be collected using this method. Others expressed concern over the "validity of data" since it was not derived from probability sampling techniques.

Many factors, known and unknown, contributed to ease of entry. As already described, the groundwork had been laid early; I had been employed and accepted as a staff nurse, a bona fide role which needed no further explanation. In addition, the purposes and method of the study had been discussed with physicians and nurses in administrative positions in this institution prior to seeking permission to do the study.

My identification as a nurse-sociologist served a neutralizing function in allaying suspicions of persons whose permission was required before the study could begin. Their fears of harm coming to patients were relieved when they focused on the nurse role, e.g., "but you are a nurse, so you understand what I mean." Concerns about biased reporting were quieted by focusing upon the sociologist role, e.g., "as a sociologist you will see the whole picture." Perhaps the statement made by one of these individuals said it best, "You are in a unique position to do this study, no other sociologist would be allowed in here."

Thus, from the beginning, in terms of staff members, I was to feel at the same time "insider" and "outsider." Throughout data collection, my role of researcher remained to varying degrees that of stranger, "the potential wanderer," "in" the group, but not truly "of" the group, at the same time near and far, and free to leave at any time (2).

IDENTIFICATION WITH PEOPLE STUDIED

Identifying with the people being studied allows a researcher to better understand them (3). It affords a researcher the opportunity to see the world through their eyes. At the same time, over-identification with the subjects creates the likelihood of misperception and distortion. Gans (4) states that although identification can detract from objectivity, it need not do so if researchers are consciously aware of what is happening to them.

There was the potential for over-identifying with two general groups in this study: health care providers in general, and nurses in particular; and the patients and their significant others. Several authors have indicated that a nurse in the participant observer role faces special dilemmas but has certain advantages (5). The greatest of these advantages is the background knowledge that it would take others months or years to acquire. On a more personal level, there is the advantage of less "culture shock" for an individual already accustomed to the modern medical center, its technology, and the acuity of illness of patients (6).

53

At the same time, these advantages create potential problems. A nurse may overlook relevant factors because she no longer is aware of them. Secondly, she may be faced with the dilemma of choosing between making passive objective observations as a researcher or taking the more action-oriented stance of the nurse. The dilemma of choosing between the observations of the researcher and the actions of a nurse were not a problem because both were part of the data used in the study.

I was in a unique position for purposes of this study. Although a qualified nurse, my most recent experience as a nurse had been as a faculty member in a school of nursing. In addition, the preceding three years had been spent immersed in the study of sociology. As a sociologist, I still was a nurse, but in a more abstract way. Perhaps it was an identification with the generic term nurse, but it certainly was not with a particular nursing role. The insight was gained when I was amazed when reminded by another sociologist that I was "not assuming the role of staff nurse," I was "a staff nurse."

As a researcher, I was forced to learn not only the role and duties of staff nurses in the institution, but also the relationship of staff nurses to other health care providers. Nothing could be taken for granted; I had to discover the institution's norms or common rules of behavior regarding interactions with and surrounding dying persons. In many instances, this discovery occurred when I inadvertently did not conform to an expected pattern of behavior. Although there was the common bond of "care to patients" between me and other health care providers, the differences between me and other providers reduced the dangers of over-identification with any one group. Disparities in educational background and age, and the fact that I was a part-time employee and a full-time student contributed to my status of "stranger."

Another factor which decreased the possibility of over-identification with any one group of providers or with patients and their families was the acute awareness that the successful collection of data depended upon the establishment of rapport with everyone in the situation. Although conscious of clashes in values, I was not free to confront the issue at hand. However frustrating this was at times, it served to clarify the various points of view and to produce insights useful to the study.

Although I was able to empathize with the patients and their significant others and to feel the sadness of the situation, my simultaneous roles of nurse and researcher reduced the potential for over-identification with them. However, protection from over-identification did not insulate me from feelings of ambivalence and guilt that occurred as I rendered the best care I could, while knowing that I would be analyzing these events later. This led to another problem of any participant observations study—the ethical legitimacy of the study.

ETHICAL LEGITIMACY

Questions of ethical legitimacy always have to be faced by researchers working in the natural setting. The major question addressed here is does the end justify the means.

Both patients and those interacting with them had been informed of my role as nurse-sociologist. All questions related to the dual role were answered honestly as they arose. To preserve the natural nature of the settings, no formal announcements were made to staff members regarding this study. However, my interest in the care of seriously ill and dying persons was made known. Patients and families generally were informed during the course of conversation with them. Health professionals were told directly.

The fact that friendly and professional relationships were being used for the collection of data, coupled with my feelings that these relationships were being exploited, created some conflict. However, some of these feelings of anxiety were relieved by the knowledge that the study was not directed toward malicious or harmful ends.

Safeguards did not answer the ethical question of whether the end justified the means. There was, and is, no easy answer to this problem. As a social scientist, I was attempting to describe the world as it is; and this required my observing behaviors of dying persons and others. There was no alternative; formal interviews might have been threatening to the participants and might have resulted in reports of behaviors, or attitudes toward dying, but could not provide evidence about the behaviors themselves. Not using formal interviews proved to be a sound decision. Observing and listening to patients and those interacting with them revealed answers to questions I would not have thought to ask. Questions on sensitive subjects were asked only as deemed appropriate in the context of the entire interaction and then only when I perceived my relationship with the person as being well enough established to allow such questioning. In brief, I attempted to prevent any unnecessary emotional trauma to the subjects as a result of the study.

ANALYZING THE DATA

Data analysis consisted primarily of classification of data to identify patterns, qualities, or processes which typify the situation of and surrounding the hospitalized dying person. In essence, it was a matter of categorizing data to describe the dynamics or stages of change in meanings and interactional relationships.

The transcribed field notes of observations, conversations, impressions, data from medical and nursing records, and demographic data on each subject constituted the data for analysis. Photocopies of field notes were made to facilitate categorizing the data. Categorizations were determined by the initial research objective, sensitizing concepts and questions, and through additional discoveries made while in the field. In addition, a case study was compiled on each subject. Case studies consisted of (1) a patient profile, which included a description of the patient and his or her perceptions of life and illness; (2) a social history, including life-style and economic and emotional support systems; (3) a medical history including past and present illnesses as well as course of present illness; (4) a medical assessment and therapeutic regimen; and (5) a nursing assessment and nursing regimen.

The data were analyzed to identify themes and patterns which answered the major questions of this study. For example, to explore the question, *Is the initial label of dying socially defined and differentially applied?*, the data were reread and examined to ascertain at what place in time and under what circumstances a label was applied and by whom. These data were also reviewed to explore *when and under what circumstances a label was accepted for use and by whom.* Sources of data, such as interactions with patients and family members, medical records, nursing care plans, change of shift reports, and physicians' reports provided differing perspectives at the same place in time and over time. These differences were essential to exploring the above question and the closely related question, namely, *What is the process leading to a common definition of a situation, where the parameters are either unknown or taboo?* Data were analyzed to identify factors which contributed to or detracted from a common definition. For instance, one factor observed as influencing the process was the pattern of communication between and among interactors.

In exploring the question, *How are roles formed under conditions of relative normlessness?*, it was necessary first to determine if there were norms or rules governing behavior in the situation. The data were analyzed first to identify these norms. The possible effects of social factors, such as social class, age, sex, and previous experiences with death were then analyzed in regard to each major question.

Social class was determined by using the Hollingshead Two Factor Index of Social Position (7) which is based on the occupation and education of the head of household. In all instances, the occupation considered to be primary by the subject was used in determining social position. This resulted in a greater number of persons being classified at the upper end of the index. Many of these individuals were either temporarily or permanently unemployed because of illness or retirement. In some instances the subjects' illness made it necessary for them to assume positions of lesser responsibility and status.

A cross-sectional analysis was done to present a general description of the complexity of the situation and to provide a portrait of the dying person and the interactors. This retrospective analysis was done at the completion of data collection, quantifying characteristics wherever possible.

Statistical tests were not appropriate for use with this data nor would they add to the findings, thus no statistical analysis was done. The findings from the retrospective analysis are described in the next chapter.

REFERENCES

1. Filstead W: Qualitative Methodology: Firsthand Involvement with the Social World, Chicago, Markham Publishing Co., 1970, especially pp. 1 – 11; McCall G, Simmons JL (eds): Issues in Participant Observation: A Text and Reader, Reading, Mass., Addison-Wesley Publishing Co., 1969, especially preface
2. Simmel G: The stranger. *In* Wolff KH (ed): The Sociology of Georg Simmel, New York, The Free Press, 1950, pp. 402 – 08
3. Lofland J: Analyzing Social Settings, a Guide to Qualitative Observation and Analysis, Belmont, Calif., Wadsworth Publishing Company, Inc., 1971, pp. 1 – 3; Berger P, Luckman T: The Social Construction of Reality: A Treatise in the Sociology of Knowledge, New York, Doubleday Co., 1967, especially pp. 28 – 34; Schutz A: The Phenomenology of the Social World, Evanston, Ill., Northwestern University Press, 1967, especially Chapter 4, Sections C and D
4. Gans H: The Urban Villagers: Group and Class in the Life of Italian-Americans, New York, The Free Press, 1962, p. 242
5. Poulos ES, McCabe GS: The nurse in the role of research observer. Nurs Res, 9 (Summer 1960), pp. 137 – 140; Malone M: The research nurse and social science research. *In*

Bennis WC et al: The Role of the Nurse in the Outpatient Department, New York, American Nurses Foundation, 1961, pp. 86 – 88

6. Pearsall M: Participant observation as role and method in behavioral research. *In* Qualitative Methodology: Firsthand Involvement with the Social World, Chicago, Markham Publishing Company, 1970, pp. 340 – 52

7. Hollingshead AB: Two Factor Index of Social Position (Unpublished manuscript), 1965 Yale Station, New Haven, Conn., 1957

5 The Interactors and the Interactional Milieu

A description of the interactors in the study and the interactional milieu provides some insight into the complexity of the situation of which the patient and his family became an integral part. A detailed description of the social setting and organizational structure serves as the background for all interactions. It includes an analysis of the influence of the environment upon the professionals involved in the care of the dying patients. The major portion of the chapter describes the patients and their families.

THE INTERACTIONAL MILIEU

The study was conducted in a large midwestern medical center whose stated purposes are patient care, education, and research. It is a tertiary care, referral facility which provides intensive care and treatment for people with acute and complex health problems which cannot be treated in other hospitals. This medical center focuses upon cure and achieving the optimum level of comfort and function for individual patients. It is not specifically designed for the care of chronically ill or dying patients. Admission to this institution may imply a high level of acuity of illness; it does not define the patient as dying.

ORGANIZATIONAL STRUCTURE AND INTERACTIONAL RELATIONSHIPS

The organizational structure of a hospital contributes both to the type of care a patient receives during the course of an illness and to the degree of autonomy available to patients and other interactors. Autonomy was especially important in this study because options for behavior of patients and other interactors are influenced by the degree of autonomy available to each within the pre-existing structure.

When people are admitted to a hospital they are introduced into a pre-existing *group* comprised of nurses, physicians, other care providers, and other patients. Patients are usually admitted to a hospital for the treatment of an illness or, if an illness is untreatable, for relief from discomfort, which becomes the goal of the health care providers. Patients, family, and health care providers may have differing and conflicting views about means necessary to achieve a cure or relieve discomfort.

The group members participate in pre-established roles and role relationships to perform tasks essential to the control of ills and to maintain comfort. These tasks and goals influence all interactional relationships. They do not, however, explicitly define behaviors related to interacting with dying patients, nor do they eliminate conflict among the various interactors.

Usually many persons are involved in the care of a patient: physicians, nurses, therapists, technicians, social workers, clergy, students of medicine and nursing, and hospital administrators, as well as family or friends who may interact with the patient who is hospitalized. These persons play different but related roles. Patients and their families commonly interact with several members of the group during a hospital stay. Since the major day-to-day interactions occur in areas where patients are housed, the majority of interactions are with personnel assigned to these patient care units. Behavioral expectations and relationships primarily develop during and as a result of interactions.

The interactional relationships and channels of communication of those directly responsible for the care of patients on a patient care unit are depicted in Figure 1, which is a simplified model of the complexity of interactions that are possible. It represents interactions regarding one patient, the family, and visitors.

A three-dimensional model would be more representative, including any number of patients and families who interact with each other, and with the depicted health care providers and others. Patients, their families, and other visitors play a primary role in socializing other patients and their families and visitors into the hospital's system. Patients interact most frequently with their families and their patient-roommates and next most frequently with nurses and nursing personnel.

In Figure 1, nursing support staff includes licensed practical nurses, nursing aides, unit managers, and unit secretaries. Nurse refers to registered nurses who are responsible for and participate in direct patient care.

The term house officers refers to interns and residents who are licensed physicians furthering their education and practicing medicine under the supervision of experienced licensed physicians.

AUTONOMY AND HIERARCHICAL STRUCTURE

As mentioned, autonomy is an important factor in role relations. It is enhanced by the organizational structure of this hospital. Figure 1 implicitly depicts the hierarchical structure of this hospital.

In this setting there are three parallel hierarchical, policy-making structures: hospital administration, medical council, and nursing council. Both the School of Nursing and School of Medicine are closely aligned with the hospital and influence both the policies and practices of their respective professions. Hospital administration assumes responsibility for fiscal concerns, management of all support services, and personnel policies. Thus, there is a nursing hierarchy, a medical hierarchy, and a hospital administrative hierarchy with formalized channels of communication between and among the various levels.

Matters of joint concern are considered together. Recommendations are then made with each council responsible for having policies implemented through appropriate channels.

There is no intent to imply equal status or lack of conflict between members of nursing and medical councils, or between individual physicians and nurses. The lack of a representative from the Board of Trustees on the nursing council may reflect the differences in status accorded to physicians and to nurses by this body.

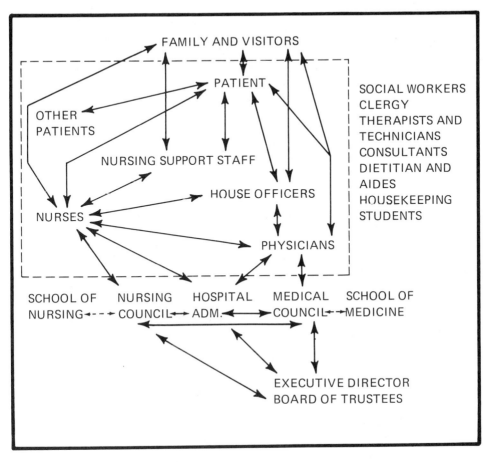

Figure 1. — Interactional Relationships and Communication.

Arrows represent interactional relationships and channels of communication. Those people within the boundary lines commonly interact on a daily basis. People outside these lines interact with patients and others on the unit periodically.

POLICIES FOR PRACTICE

All policies and guidelines for nursing practice are in written form, available on each patient care unit, and can be consulted at any time. There are role descriptions which define expectations for each type of nursing personnel. These include general expectations defining types of activities (such as primary assessment of patients' problems). There are no explicit rules or regulations governing interactional relationships. Decisions regarding behavior or actions in any given situation are based upon individual judgments. The formal organizational structure provides a framework rather than specific and well-delineated regulations for behavior.

The goals of the hospital remained the same over the time that the data were collected. Individual and group judgments were shared verbally and dictated specific behaviors used to achieve goals. In most instances, judgments were influenced by the characteristics of the professional groups, nursing and medicine, and the criteria each used to evaluate a situation. Individual physicians and nurses viewed the situation from their own hierarchical position and ideological stance. Conflict was inherent in many situations. A brief review of the characteristics of each group may lend further insight into their respective positions and behaviors.

THE INTERACTORS

REGISTERED NURSES AND NURSING PERSONNEL

The characteristics of the nurses caring for patients on the 36-bed medical patient care unit were similar to those of the nurses on the 13-bed surgical intensive care unit. Thirteen of the 15 registered nurses on the medical unit had baccalaureate degrees in nursing, one was a graduate of a diploma program, and one registered nurse position was filled by five part-time nurses: one with an M.S.N. degree, two with B.S.N. degrees, and two with diplomas. In addition to the 15 registered nurses, there were eight licensed practical nurses and three nurses' aides.

The surgical intensive care unit was staffed by 25 registered nurses. The nurse in charge had an M.S.N. degree; 18 of the registered nurses had B.S.N. degrees; and five were graduates of diploma schools of nursing. Three of the five diploma graduates were engaged in part-time study toward a B.S.N. degree. The remaining registered nurse was an associate degree graduate who had worked for many years as a licensed practical nurse prior to earning an associate degree in nursing. Four licensed practical nurses and three nurses' aides were also assigned to the surgical intensive care unit.

Although the nurses and nursing personnel varied somewhat in terms of their personal approach to patients, they had a common commitment to individualized patient care. Written plans of care (see Appendix) for individual patients illustrate the attempt to individualize the nursing care of each patient. Some commonalities were evident in nursing care plans, reports, conversations, and nursing actions. These commonalities reflected the values of these nurses in caring for dying patients. The most evident common values were the rights of patients to know their diagnoses and prognoses; to participate in making informed decisions regarding their nursing and medical care for as long as they were able; and the right to die with dignity.

The most striking observable factor about the registered nurses was their youth. All were under age 30 with the mean age being 24 years. Their work experience ranged from zero to five years following graduation from their respective schools of nursing. In contrast, the licensed practical nurses and aides were at least a decade older than the registered nurses and had more years of experience in caring for patients. All of them had been employed by this hospital for more than seven years.

HOUSE OFFICERS: RESIDENTS AND INTERNS

The house officers shared similar educational backgrounds, three to four years of college and four years of medical school. Most were under 30 years of age. Generally, there were two residents and two interns assigned to the medical unit for a three- to four-month rotation. The residents were responsible for the medical care of their assigned patients as well as for teaching and supervising the interns. The medical coverage of the surgical intensive care unit was more varied. Three house officers were assigned to the intensive care unit for a three- or four-month rotation. In addition, there were many resident house officers who served as consultants.

The expressed views of the house officers toward the patients varied. Their interactions and decisions reflected, in most instances, the philosophy and attitudes of the patient's private physician. Their short stay on a unit and their desire to learn as much as possible while there contributed to their focus on their own individual learning interests which sometimes took precedence over the needs and desires of patients.

PRIVATE PHYSICIANS

There were 29 private physicians responsible for the care of patients in this study. They were predominantly specialists in their own fields (hematology, cardiology, oncology, internal medicine, and surgery). They were the oldest and most experienced of the health care providers. Their views regarding the rights of patients varied widely. The majority told patients their *diagnoses* directly but, in most cases, patients were not directly informed about their *prognoses.*

VISITORS: FAMILY AND SIGNIFICANT OTHERS

Policies and Practices. Both hospital policy and actions of health care providers encouraged visiting. Visiting hours were from 8:00 a.m. to 8:00 p.m. on the medical and from 9:00 a.m. to 9:00 p.m. on the surgical intensive care unit. The number of visitors at any one time and the length of a visit depended upon the acuity of illness, needed therapeutic intervention, and the wishes of patients and their roommates. When conflicts arose, the nurse in charge of the unit usually made the final decision regarding the number of visitors and the length of visits. Visiting hours were not rigidly enforced on either unit. When patients were critically ill, families were allowed to stay in the patient's room or in the adjoining waiting room 24 hours a day.

The majority of patients actively participated for as long as they were able in deciding whether or not they wanted visitors. Their participation did not guarantee that people would or would not visit, or that the people who visited would be individuals the patient would most like to see. Most patients continued to welcome short visits of five to twenty minutes from significant others throughout their illness. Patients expressed their regret when visitors no longer came and remorse when they no longer received cards or telephone calls.

Generally, during long or repeated admissions, only close relatives or friends continued to visit. The decrease in visitors occurred even when the patients were physically able and desirous of visits from other friends, relatives, and associates.

Most patients and their families expressed regret and feelings of isolation and loneliness when friends and associates no longer visited.

Patients and family members generally welcomed conversations with strangers, including other patients, as well as the visitors of other patients. Many patients and family members established lasting relationships during these conversations. It was common to have former patients and their families visit or inquire about other patients and their families.

In three situations patients questioned the motives of a relative for visiting and shared their feelings and observations with me and other nurses. These patients believed the visits were more prompted by the visitors' feelings of guilt, morbid curiosity, and their need to impress others, especially the nurses, than out of concern for them. They commented that the relative had not expressed concern about them, contacted them, or visited them at home or in the hospital during prior admissions. Further, in their view, the only reason the relatives visited at all was because they thought the patient would die soon.

Whether or not patients questioned the intent of visitors, they welcomed them, thanked them for coming, and invited them to come again. All three patients refused my offer and the offer of other nurses to intervene and suggest that the visitors leave and allow the patient to rest. When the visitors did leave, the patients once again became visibly upset and expressed to me and other nurses their anger and wishes that the visitors would not come again.

Members of the patient's immediate family or close friends exerted influence over who visited the patient. Usually physicians informed a family member (generally parents or spouse) or a close friend, if family were not available, of the critical nature of the patient's condition. The informed person(s) decided how, where, by whom, when, whether or how much, if any, information would be shared with the patient and others (children, friends, or other relatives). Informed individuals were in a position to directly and indirectly control the access of others to the patients through the type of information they disseminated.

Patients generally welcomed having a family member or close friend nearby, if not at their bedside. The visitors sat quietly at the patient's bedside, reading or occupying themselves with puzzles or handiwork, or sat in the corridors or in the waiting room. Patients enjoyed intermittently talking with visitors, napping, or sharing the quiet presence of another person.

Family Members and Patterns of Visits. Although there was great variation in the characteristics of the patients' visitors, some discernible visiting patterns were observed. Members of the patient's immediate family were the most consistent visitors. This was an anticipated finding since our society perceives the family as being responsible for the care of its members either directly or indirectly. Even when others no longer visited, family members had no recourse. The ultimate responsibility for the patient was theirs, whether or not they wanted it or felt able to cope with it. They handled the situation in differing ways but all were bound by emotional, social, economic, and legal obligations.

Age and marital status were associated with differences in patterns of visiting. For the 19 patients who were 48 years old or younger, their parents or spouse were the primary visitors. Three of these patients were unmarried teenagers. Their parents visited almost constantly, at times alternating their visits so that one could attend to other responsibilities while the other was present in the hospital.

In this age group, 14 of the subjects were married. In about half of these cases, visiting was a cooperative effort between the spouse, parents, and parents-in-law. Usually, the spouse, whether male or female, was the central figure with parents offering advice, support, and assistance. In cases of unmarried patients, parents became central to interactions. Siblings and, less frequently, colleagues also offered assistance.

The pattern of visiting was somewhat different for 19 subjects between the ages of 49 and 75. The spouses assumed major responsibility for the 12 married subjects. They were occasionally accompanied by their children, but more frequently were alone or with friends. Parents of this age group were often aged, disabled, living out of town, or deceased. Those who visited usually came on weekends. Frequently there were long telephone conversations between patients (women usually) and their parents.

In some instances, patients' children assumed responsibility for the home and for younger children. In other instances, children were living out of town. For whatever reasons, children were not consistently present, although they maintained contact throughout their parent's illness. When death was viewed as imminent within days, children visited more regularly and frequently. Two of these patients wished to die at home and were discharged to the homes of their children to fulfill their wish.

There were four widowed patients in this age group. They relied predominantly upon siblings and children for visits. Two of them had been living with their siblings and two had been living with their children before admission to the hospital.

There were no observed differences in visiting patterns related to social position with the exception that patients of the professional strata, especially unmarried patients, were more consistently visited by colleagues than members of any other strata. They also relied upon colleagues rather than upon family members more frequently than members of other social positions.

Of the nine patients between the ages of 79 and 88, three were married and their spouses were consistently present. Although friends, neighbors, nieces, and nephews visited the other six patients occasionally, they were alone most of the time. In two instances, their children were present consistently during the afternoons and evenings. Of the other six patients, five were widowed and one man had never been married. Two of the six relied upon their nieces for biweekly visits. One 84-year-old woman had no living relatives and was only occasionally visited by an elderly neighbor.

In general, the nine patients between the ages of 79 and 88 had few persons available to visit them. Most of their friends and siblings had died or were unable to come to the hospital to see them.

THE PATIENTS

Age, Sex, and Life Status.   Forty-seven patients, 30 women and 17 men, constituted the primary focus for observation. Five were patients on the surgical intensive care unit, and 42 were patients on the medical unit.

Seventeen of the 30 women died during the period of the study. The women ranged in age from 23 to 88 years, with a mean of 56.6 years and a median of 49 years. Fifteen of the women died in the hospital, one died at home, and one died in a nursing home. The 13 women living at the end of data collection ranged in age from 28 to 87 years, with a mean of 53.7 years and a median of 60 years. The age range for the total sample of women was the same as for those who died, but the mean age was lower, 54.8 years, and the median age higher, 58 years.

The 17 men in the study ranged in age from 14 to 85 years, with a mean age of 48 and a median of 50 years. Two of these men, ages 31 and 32, were alive at the completion of data collection, and both were hospitalized.

The mean age at the time of death for the 15 men who died was 50.2 with a median of 59 years. Two of the men died at home and the other 13 died in the hospital. The mean age at death was lowered because it included two 14-year-old boys. Excluding these subjects, the mean age at death for males would have been 55.8 (see Table 1).

The subjects, regardless of sex, died at a comparatively young age. According to the U.S. Bureau of Census, the national projected life expectancy in the United States in 1974 was 75.2 years for women and 67.4 for men. Thus, as might be expected in a study about dying, many patients died younger than the projected life expectancy. Death at these young ages was related to the pathophysiological problems of these individuals, and the nature of admissions to this medical center.

Diagnoses. Patients are described in terms of general categories such as cancer or cardiovascular disease rather than specific diagnoses such as specific types of cancer (lymphosarcoma, or oat cell carcinoma of the lung); or specific cardiovascular problems (such as anteriolateral myocardial infarct or coronary artery thrombosis). The intent is to present a broad picture of the types of illnesses experienced by subjects rather than to address issues related to any particular disease entities. Large diagnostic categories include treatable as well as non-treatable problems. None of these categories, including cancers, is synonymous with death. The course of illness and prognosis rather than a particular diagnostic label are of greater importance in this study because the process of dying superseded the uniqueness of any diagnosis. In general, people whose

Table 1.—Summary: Sex, Age in Years, and Status of Patients at Completion of Data Collection (N = 47).

Sex and Status	Number	Mean Age	Age Range
Women			
Living	13	53.7	28 — 87
Died	17	56.6	23 — 88
TOTAL	30	54.8	23 — 88
Men			
Living	2	31.5	31 — 32
Died	15	50.2	14 — 85
TOTAL	17	48	14 — 85

Table 2.—Diagnostic Category by Mean Age, Status, and
Sex at Completion of Data Collection (N = 47).

	Cancers and Malignant Diseases				Other Disease Conditions			
	Alive		Died		Alive		Died	
	f	$\bar{x}$ age	f	$\bar{x}$ age	f	$\bar{x}$ age	f	$\bar{x}$ age
Women	12	55.2	11	47.3	1	87	6	73.8
Men	1	35	8	49.1	1	31	7	51.4*
TOTAL	13		19		2		14	

*Excluding the two 14-year-olds, the mean age was 66.4 years; f = frequency; $\bar{x}$ = mean.

death occurred during this study had in common the fact that their illnesses did not respond to available therapies.

Thirty-two of the subjects had cancers and other forms of malignant disease. Of the seven individuals with vascular diseases, two had cerebrovascular disease and five had cardiovascular disease. Two persons had hepatic disease, and three pulmonary disorders. One 14-year-old boy died of sepsis and one as a result of an accident. Table 2 depicts the living status of men and women, their mean ages, and their diagnostic categories.

Hospitalization and Hospital Days. For the majority of the 47 patients, illness and hospitalization were not strangers. Nearly all experienced multiple hospital admissions, many days confinement to the hospital, or both. One-quarter were directly transferred to this institution from other hospitals. About one-half had been hospitalized in other institutions at some time during the course of their illness.

The length of illness for the persons who died by the completion of data collection ranged from one month to four years with a mean average of ten months. Those alive at the end of data collection had been ill from one month to five years with a mean average of 30 months.

The total sample accounted for over 200 separate admissions to the medical center during the two years of data collection. The average number of admissions was five, with the range being from two to 28. The admissions totaled over 2,000 hospital days, averaging approximately 50 days per person. The range was from two to over 200 hospital days per person. Consecutive days of confinement varied from as few as two to over 100 days per person. The figures are at best conservative. They include only admissions to and hospital stays in the medical center and include only admissions related to illness which eventually led to the person's dying status.

The number of hospital confinement days, in particular consecutive confinement days, was an important factor in the study. During short stays of one week or less, interactions were on an impersonal level and were focused on the treatment of physical symptomatology and completion of diagnostic tests. Interactors followed the prescribed rules of behavior generally attributed to their formal roles. There was little time spent in negotiating for modified roles or in gaining insight into each other's definition of the situation.

Building of relationships occurred over time. Multiple short stays on the same unit and interaction with the same care givers provided opportunities for negotiation, development of roles, and consensus about what was going on in terms of the patients' health status. Consecutive hospital stays from approximately two to five weeks had the same results. There was a point of diminishing returns, however. With stays of longer than five consecutive weeks interactions decreased, the situation coalesced, and all the interactors appeared perplexed as to how to terminate the relationship, especially when the patient's condition neither improved nor deteriorated.

It is not possible to determine from the data exact parameters of how long a stay is most conducive to developing positive relationships. Further study is needed to identify more exact parameters.

Another variable which affected interactions was the patterns of living-dying which culminated in death.

PATTERNS OF LIVING-DYING

A retrospective analysis of the data revealed four major patterns of living-dying (Figure 2) which culminated in death. These will be referred to as: (1) Peaks and Valleys, (2) Descending Plateaus, (3) Downward Slopes, and (4) Gradual Slants.*

The patterns of living-dying are included here for descriptive purposes. It is premature and inappropriate to use them clinically in a prospective or predictive fashion. Their importance will become more apparent as the major questions of the study are discussed in later chapters. The patterns were identified by examining the patients' life from the time they first became subjects until data collection was completed or the patient died.

Peaks and Valleys. This pattern of living-dying was characterized by periods of crisis and periods of quiescence, or what is commonly referred to as exacerbations and remissions. Patients refer to these as "hopeful highs" and "terrible" or "depressing lows." This pattern can be conceptualized as a series of erratic peaks and valleys, with the peaks representing periods of greater health (remissions) and the valleys, times of crisis (exacerbations) with increased signs and symptoms of pathology. Individuals with this pattern had multiple admissions to the hospital, predominantly occurring during the periods of crisis. Both the heights of the peaks and the depths of the valleys were indeterminate in time as was the duration of remaining at any point. There was an overriding downward slope. The peaks became progressively less high, but the valleys did not necessarily become lower, though the valleys did last for increasingly longer periods of time.

Although there are diseases characterized by periods of remission and exacerbation, such as the leukemias, this pattern was not specific to any disease classification. It was a pattern of living-dying, as were the others, which was not necessarily related to the natural pathology of any disease classification. Periods

---

*Although not manifested in this study, it is conceivable that many combinations of these patterns could be identified if the study were replicated with different populations of subjects (e.g., ambulatory, well aged, children) in differing environments (e.g., nursing homes, rehabilitation centers, hospices, homes).

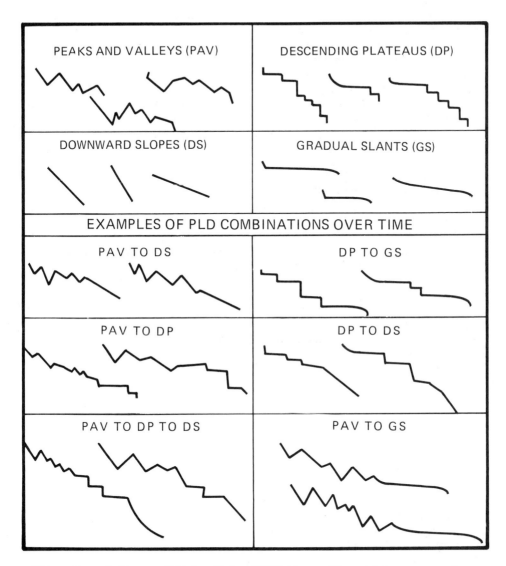

Figure 2. — Patterns of Living-Dying (PLD): Some Pictorial Representations.

Theoretically many combinations could be illustrated. The examples are those identified by Sr. Karin Dufault in her research, "Hope and Elderly Persons with Cancer" (unpublished doctoral dissertation, School of Nursing, Case Western Reserve University, Cleveland, Ohio, in progress, used with permission). Unlike the present study, these patterns of living which culminated in death evolved over a period of weeks to as many as sixteen years.

of remission in many instances were related to medical interventions rather than to the natural course of disease.

The peaks and valleys pattern of living-dying was associated with uncertainties for all concerned. It was difficult for the interactors to determine whether their emphasis should be on plans for living or for dying. At times, no one (health care providers, family members, or patients) could predict what the next day would bring. Raised hopes gave way to disappointments. At other times, just as patients and family members became resigned to the probability of a patient's death, there would be a remission. Even when remissions became improbable and all available medical therapies had failed, family members and patients clung to the hope of another remission. They cited past experiences to support these hopes. Health care providers sometimes supported these hopes, usually through their silence, and at other times attempted to dispel them. Uncertainty and ambiguity was increased when at the same time some health care providers supported the possibility of remission and others negated it.

Descending Plateaus. Another common pattern was that of progressive degenerative plateaus occurring an unpredictable number of times and for indeterminate periods of time. In these cases the individual continued on a relatively stable course until some crisis intervened. There was recovery from the crisis but not return to the former level of health or functional ability. This pattern can be depicted as a series of steps in which the heights may vary as may the duration of the plateaus.

Like the peaks and valley patterns, this pattern was characterized by an element of uncertainty. The uncertainty was related to whether or when another crisis might occur causing further debilitation. Associated with it were expressions of anger, depression, and futility by patients and family over the loss of functional ability after concerted rehabilitative efforts.

Downward Slopes. The third pattern was that of continuous downward slopes. In this pattern, the degree of the slope represented acuity of illness and the length of the slope represented the duration of illness. Although the slopes differed in degree and length, there was a persistent, consistent, and easily discernible downward course. In general, these individuals had shorter duration of illness antecedent to death than individuals with any of the other patterns.

Under the conditions of usually sudden, persistent, and rapid degeneration of health, interactions became more intense. Interactions were predominantly limited to health care providers who focused primarily on possible medical and nursing interventions to maintain life. Patients usually were physically unable to actively participate in any decisions about their care. Family members were called on when permission was needed to institute new treatment modalities, including extraordinary means to sustain life.

Generally, health care providers focused on the immediate care of the patient. They did not consistently keep family members informed of the patient's health status during the period of crisis. When a crisis abated or the patient died, more extensive reports were shared with family members. Generally, interactions were short and intense and there was little or no time for patients or family members to prepare for the death.

Gradual Slants. The fourth pattern of living-dying was the gradual slant. This pattern is depicted by an almost continuous low ebb of life, gradually and sometimes almost imperceptibly culminating in death. In general, individuals exhibiting this pattern experienced a major debilitating bodily insult. They were apt to have fewer total hospital admissions than individuals with either the plateaus or peaks and valleys patterns. Moreover, they were likely to be hospitalized in other facilities such as nursing homes or chronic care centers. This pattern was either long or short in terms of duration of time preceding the death event.

A series of problems was associated with patients living for prolonged periods with this pattern. When known therapies were exhausted and death was imminent, yet the patient continued to survive, questions were raised regarding definitions of death. Is the person alive when there is no brain function but the heart continues to beat? Moral and legal questions arose. Should respirators be discontinued although breathing, and thus living, might cease? Would discontinuing ineffective therapy constitute euthanasia? Under the described conditions, do modern technologies prolong living or dying? Placement of patients was another problem especially associated with the gradual slants pattern. When known therapies were exhausted and no improvement in the patients' physical status occurred, where should patients be cared for, and who should be responsible for their care?

Social position, ethnicity, and religion were other characteristics of subjects that influenced interactions.

SOCIAL POSITION

Social position was based upon occupation and education of the head of household, usually husband or father. The social position of single (never married, separated, divorced, widowed) adults over age 21 was determined by their own education and occupation. Since the majority of subjects was unemployed by completion of data collection, the occupation they considered as primary was used.

The reported educational experience of subjects ranged from less than eight years of schooling to the completion of graduate and professional schools. Occupations were varied, ranging from unskilled laborers to major professionals and executives of large businesses or concerns.

The scores were skewed toward the upper end of the continuum, using Hollingshead's five position hierarchy. The groups were collapsed for descriptive purposes into Professional (Groups 1 and 2—16 subjects), White Collar (Groups 3 and 4—14 subjects), and Blue Collar (Group 5—7 subjects). The social position of three men and seven women was not determined because either occupation, education, or both were not obtained.

Educational background generally was not discussed during casual conversation. Three subjects who had completed greater than four years of college referred to their former intellectual achievement as a standard for evaluating their present intellectual abilities and activities. There were such comments as "I used to answer all the questions on quiz shows, now I can't understand the questions," or "I was the first in my class in graduate school, it's one thing when your body goes, but when your mind . . . there will be nothing left of me."

References to formal education also were made in combination with references to past employment. Once the subjects initiated these topics they generally elaborated on them, often tracing the paths of their own work careers and that of their spouse or family members. In most instances they talked of their former prowess, whether physical or intellectual, or if talking about a family member, their own contributions to the family member's educational or employment successes.

Educational background, social activities, and employment served as both indicators for evaluating physical and intellectual status and as means for maintaining a personal identity divorced from that of *patient*. It was important to patients and family members that the patients maintain their identity as attractive, productive, human beings. Pictures of patients prior to their illnesses frequently were shared with other interactors, as were reports of awards or honors. There are many ways to interpret these conversations and sharing of memorabilia. One interpretation, of importance in interacting with dying patients, is the attempt to establish a common bond with the health care providers and others. A bond which says "I am dying, or I am ill, but I am a person. I am not different, I am like you." This bonding theme became more apparent when looking at other characteristics which patients had in common with other interactors. Common ethnic background was such a characteristic.

RACE AND ETHNICITY

The sample was predominantly white, but included two black subjects, both of whom were female. Five people identified themselves as Irish, six as Jewish, one as Hungarian, one as Polish, one as English, one as German, and seven as Italian.

The patients who identified themselves as Italian, Irish, and German often used this information as a means of opening conversation with me, when they recognized my name as being Italian in origin. I repeatedly was told, "You're Italian so you will understand." Others spoke of their ethnic backgrounds in relation to religious holidays and food preferences.

RELIGION AND RELIGIOUSNESS

Information about religion and religiousness was obtained through observation and by listening to the comments of patients and their families. All references to religion were initiated by patients or families. I made no attempt to ask direct questions about religion, religious beliefs, or interest and participation in religious activities.

All patients' rooms had bedside stands, and bulletin boards which patients could decorate as they wished. More than half of the subjects had religious items displayed in their rooms or on their persons. Sometimes patients requested these items, at other times they received them as gifts. Most patients made a point of telling me about them, but some made no mention of them.

Religious preference was obtained from the hospital admission form since I believed that asking patients their religious preference might have affected the nature of the nurse-patient interaction. It is possible that patients who mentioned neither religion nor religious beliefs, and did not display religious items, entertained religious thoughts. It is also possible that they prayed in private and followed religious tenets for behavior. However, there is no way to determine from the data whether this was so.

Timing and Incidents of Religious Content. Regardless of stated religious preference, length of hospital stay or patterns of living-dying, patients rarely initiated discussions of religious or metaphysical beliefs, or displayed religious items early in their illnesses, perhaps because they were not asked. Of the total sample, only two people, both women, referred to religion early in their illnesses.

One woman was Catholic, of Italian descent, and a member of the blue-collar class. She had symptoms of fatigue and fever and was admitted for diagnostic tests. She was extremely frightened that she had leukemia and would die as her sister had three years previously. Her physician suspected that she did have leukemia. He had known her for many years and described her as a person "who liked to worry about her worries." Although she did not openly discuss religious beliefs, each night she slept with her rosary beads wrapped tightly about her fingers. Her reliance upon religious beliefs on admission was neither encouraged nor discouraged by physicians or nurses. Data did not reveal why physicians and nurses did not attend to the spiritual aspects of her care. In past years some professionals considered it inappropriate to discuss private opinions about controversial subjects such as religion or politics with patients. Perhaps in this instance nurses and physicians were unable to share their own beliefs. Some professionals may have believed that the patient would interpret the mention of spiritual matters as an indicator that her illness was severe and her prognosis grave.

The second woman, a member of the professional class, was also Catholic and of Italian descent. She had extensive medical knowledge and had had personal experiences with others who had died of the same illness. To the question "Is there anything more I can do to make you comfortable?" she responded, "That is between God and me." Again, this initial statement was accepted by nurses and physicians at face value with neither encouragement nor discouragement, but the nurses and physicians appeared uncomfortable with her. Once outside the room, the nurses and physicians expressed their discomfort to each other. The nurses suggested the possibility of notifying a priest, but the physicians suggested that it was too early in the patient's illness for this.

Many of the nurses and physicians did not perceive spiritual care as within their realm of practice unless death was imminent within hours or days. Even then, many saw it more properly as relegated to members of the clergy or other religious. As the hour of death drew closer, this woman's references to God increased. The nurses, as well as her family, encouraged her to rely upon her religious beliefs and practices. They prayed with her and made certain her rosary beads were within reach. I observed this change of pattern from tacit acceptance of religious comments to encouragement of reliance upon the dying person's and family's religious practices when death was perceived as probable within days by the dying person, family, friends, or health care providers.

In over one-third of the patients, symbols of religious beliefs or reaching out to the metaphysical for explanations and assistance became overt within days or hours preceding death. Ten of these 12 patients were women. One exception was a young Jewish professional man who requested that a religious item be pinned to his bulletin board. He had end-stage renal disease and frequently expressed the wish to die. Neither he nor any other interactors perceived his death as imminent within days or even weeks.

73

The pattern of expressing religious beliefs immediately preceding the event of death did not vary with the type of religious orientation. Approximately half of the patients of each religious preference made reference to religious beliefs or had religious items in their rooms or on their persons prior to death.

Fourteen of the 17 Catholic patients were dead by the completion of data collection. Six of these made reference to religious beliefs or had religious items (e.g., statues, rosary beads, pictures) on display. Of the 16 patients who stated their religious preference as Protestant, 10 were dead by the end of data collection. Five of them displayed items of a religious nature, usually pictures.

Two of the six Jewish patients died during data collection. One of these patients prayed to die and had a mezuzah pinned to her bulletin board. Since she had no family, she asked me to say the following prayer immediately following the moment of death. She carefully printed the prayer with the markings and the omission of the letter "o" in God.

Shḿa Yisroal ahhdónoy
ehlóhanu, ahhdónoy ehchad.

Hear O Israel, The Lord Our G-d,
The Lord is One.

All four patients who omitted reference to any religious preference were dead by completion of data collection. Two of these patients were comatose for three to four days immediately preceding death. Their families were present, but made no mention of religious beliefs, nor did they bring religious items to the hospital. The other two patients were able to speak until shortly before death, but they made no reference to religion or religious beliefs.

Two of the four patients who specifically stated they had no religion died. They displayed no indicators of religious orientation, made no reference to religious beliefs, or any form of afterlife.

Religious Beliefs, a Taboo Subject. The findings of this study regarding religion and religious beliefs are inconclusive, limited and, at best, provide a conservative estimate of the importance of religion and religious beliefs to people during the many crises they experienced throughout the course of their illnesses. Systematic study is necessary to draw any definitive conclusion, but some observations are of importance.

Religion and religious beliefs, like dying and death, are taboo topics of conversation for many people. Some health care providers, especially physicians and nurses, described discussions of religion and religious beliefs as too personal, too revealing, and as an invasion of patients' privacy. Other health care providers stated that discussions of religion were inappropriate, especially in the scientific setting of the medical center. Many health care providers believed that religion should be discussed only when death was imminent, and that if patients wish to discuss religion, health care providers should take the passive role of listener. All health care providers felt religious beliefs of patients were important. The majority seemed unclear regarding their own role or responsibility regarding the spiritual needs of patients, other than to mention contacting a member of clergy.

In situations where there were indicators that conversations about religion or spiritual matters were acceptable and perhaps expected, such as with nursing nuns or with health care providers who either wore religious items, or who opened or invited conversations related to religion, patients discussed their religious beliefs, or lack of religious beliefs, openly throughout their illness experiences. It was usual for patients and family members to talk about their prayers and religious beliefs as sources of hope and strength.

SUMMARY

The data revealed that the situation of and surrounding the dying patients in this medical center was complex. Neither admission to the hospital nor assignment to the nursing units defined them as dying. The personnel in the hospital were bound in their activities by the single goal of achieving some "optimal level of health" for each patient. Yet, the rules that governed the behavior of personnel in achieving this goal were neither extensive nor definitive.

Nurses and physicians placed emphasis upon viewing each patient as an individual with unique problems. They believed that their actions and decisions in any situation must be based on professional judgments and tailored to patients' individual problems and therapeutic needs.

Although there was an established division of labor among health professionals based upon professional purposes, it did not remain constant. Different health professionals held different views, as did different members of the same health profession. Their views were influenced by prior experiences, as well as by their position and status in the hierarchy. The situation was further complicated by the variations in characteristics of patients and visitors, type of illness, length of hospital stay, as well as by differences in patterns of living-dying.

Roles and relationships developed among interactors during and as a result of face-to-face interactions. Conflicts between and among interactors were inherent in this dynamic situation.

Answers to the questions of: (1) how and under what circumstances is the patient defined as dying; (2) how do interactors arrive at consensus about the situation; and (3) what contributes to the evolution of varying interactor roles and relations, become more pertinent to understanding the behavior of and surrounding dying patients. These questions are addressed in Chapters 6 and 7.

6   Labels, Labeling, and Consensus

As mentioned in Chapter 3, the objective of this study was to identify qualities, patterns, and processes which typify the situation of and surrounding the dying patient in order to answer three major questions: (1) Is the label of dying socially defined? (2) How do people arrive at a common definition of the situation when the parameters are unknown, unclear, or taboo? (3) How are roles created when norms are absent, ill-defined, or conflicting?

Chapters 6 and 7 identify the processes and patterns which typify the situation surrounding the dying patient and explore the major research questions from two frames of reference, labeling and role formation. Since labeling and role formation are facets or subdivisions of the process of arriving at a common definition of the situation, discussion of the common definition is included in both chapters.

This chapter discusses what labels are used, how the label is expressed and shared, and some of the social consequences of the expression of and shared use of the labels.

The establishment of common definitions of the situation is basic to the establishment of role definitions and role relationships and they influence and are influenced by the labeling process. These questions and the underlying themes—labeling, role formation, and arrival at a common definition of the situation—are related in a reciprocal and cyclical fashion. Consequently, distinctions are analytical. Topics are discussed separately to promote understanding. The chapters and the content within the chapters are ordered to provide for clarity. There is no intent to imply a causal sequence by entering the analysis at any one phase.

LABELS AND LABELING

One of the major questions of this study was: Is the *initial* labeling of patients as dying a socially derived or biomedically defined phenomenon? Analysis of the data revealed that the question as worded did not fit empirical reality since there were actually two labels associated with individuals facing imminent death. Both of these labels were socially derived. One label was *high risk of dying** and the other label was *the dying patient.* The high risk of dying label was associated with the greater consensus than the less structured label of the dying patient.

Biomedical definitions contributed to the greater ease of application of the high risk of dying label. Patients were labeled as having a high risk of dying by virtue of their diagnostic label, guarded prognosis, or their observable physical deterioration or non-remitting progressive symptomatology. They were labeled

---

*High risk of dying is a typification, not the wording used by interactors.

as dying patients when there was common agreement that death was inevitable *within* a fairly *predictable period* of time.

The question was not whether these patients would live or die since they all were expected to die as a result of their illnesses. Although death was considered inevitable, these patients remained in the category of high risk of dying until there was consensus about the label, dying patient.

The following conversation was a key to discovering this distinction between the *high risk of dying* and the *dying patient* labels.

Mrs. N., a patient in her late eighties, was readmitted to the hospital following a third myocardial infarction. She was an alert, friendly individual, appearing much younger than her years. Although dependent upon others for most of her care, she was able to walk for short distances. She was expected to die of her heart disease, but at the same time was not considered a dying patient.

Nurse/Researcher*:	I see Mrs. N. is back again.
Nurse:	Yes, she had another infarct.
Nurse/Researcher:	Guess she won't make it.
Nurse:	(looked amazed) What do you mean, do you think she's going to die?
Nurse/Researcher:	Well, she's pretty old and had another infarct. I thought. . . . . .
Nurse: (Interrupts)	She is pretty old but she'll be okay. She'll go home again, at least this time.
Nurse/Researcher:	You don't think she is dying then?
Nurse:	Sure, she'll finally die of a heart attack or some related complication but she's not dying now. She'll go home probably a couple of times more.

It is important to understand the distinction between the *high risk of dying* and the *dying patient* from the frame of reference of those who took it for granted. Lack of understanding by any interactor leads to unnecessary conflict, accusations of dishonesty, and interpretations of lack of acceptance of death as a natural phenomenon. Health professionals might respond "no" to the question, "Are there any dying patients on this unit?" when, in fact, there were many patients in the category of *high risk of dying* but none labeled as dying per se. Persons unfamiliar with this distinction could easily misinterpret the answer as denial of reality, or an attempt to prevent access to information about patients who the questioner thought were dying. If the question were reworded to, "Do you have any patients with terminal illnesses or who aren't expected to make it?" the answer would more likely be an affirmative one. This distinction was basic to the labeling of patients and provided a starting point for arriving at a consensus about the situation. One task of the interactors, health care providers, family members, and patients was to achieve consensus about the patient's label.

---

*The term nurse/researcher is used for clarity of reporting, and to emphasize that I, the researcher, am also a nurse, whose responses and behaviors are similar to other nurses. The same or similar conversations were observed between other health care providers and patients. In all examples biographical data were altered to protect the identities of the subjects without changing the underlying meanings.

TRANSITIONAL STATES AND LABELS

There were labels other than high risk of dying and dying patient. Patients were variously labeled as well, acutely ill, chronically ill, high risk of dying, dying, and dead. These labels were applied to persons in various states of health. These states of health may be conceptualized as a continuum with a flexible and changing sequence. For example, a person could be labeled as *well*, then *acutely ill*, then *well*; or *well, high risk of dying, dying, dead*; or *high risk of dying, dying, chronically ill*; or various other combinations as depicted by the arrows in Figure 3.

Each transitional state of health had its label and associated role expectations. The boundaries were not clear and at times labels were relative. Patients with the same medical diagnosis could be labeled as acutely ill, chronically ill, high risk of dying, or dying depending upon the stability of the illness process, the emotional and physical response of the patient, and the reactions of the interactors.

There was a temporal component to all labels. A sick person was labeled as acutely ill as long as symptoms were critical, intense, or uncertain in terms of cause, treatment, or patient outcome. If recovery did not occur within a predicted duration of time or symptoms became less intense but lingered, the person was relabeled as *chronically ill*. If recovery did not occur within a predicted period of time and symptoms remained the same, the person was relabeled as *high risk of dying* or perhaps as a *dying patient*.

A re-examination of the patterns of living-dying suggests that at varying stages of each living-dying pattern, the person was labeled by interactors as *acutely ill patient, chronically ill patient*, or *high risk of dying patient* and *dying patient*. This finding suggests that labeling is a process with no one single or clearly defined sequence.

For instance, during the crisis period of the *peaks and valleys* patterns of living-dying (p. 68), the patient moved closer to the *dying* end of the continuum. During remissions they were viewed as well or chronically ill depending upon

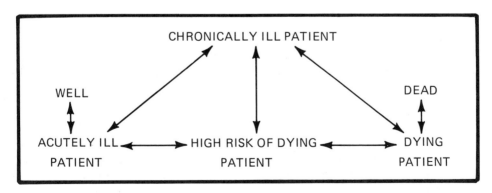

Figure 3.—Transitional States of Health.

their abilities to assume their former responsibilities and life-styles. In a like fashion, in the descending plateaus (p. 70) pattern, the patient was defined as chronically ill during plateaus. However, with increasingly progressive degeneration, they moved toward the dying patient end of the continuum. *Downward slopes* (p. 70) led most quickly and clearly to the label of dying patient while *gradual slant* patterns (p. 70) most frequently led to controversies as to whether or when patients were to be labeled as dying.

How then did a *high risk of dying* patient become the *dying* patient? Agreement about this label evolved through interactions and the sharing of information. There was *no one, well-defined point* at which the person was labeled as dying by *all* interactors *at the same time.* All interactors used their own frames of reference and cues to define the situation and arrive at the label. No single interactor was able to define the situation and impose the definition upon others. There was a process of negotiation before achieving consensus about the situation and the application of the label, *the dying patient,* occurred. In most instances the label was legitimized by common agreement. The dying patient label arose through interaction and after defining and redefining the situation. When most interactors were in agreement, the label *high risk of dying* was changed to the *dying patient.* Generally, the label was congruent with the patient's physiological status but this was not always so. In any case, the label influenced interactions.

THE DYING PATIENT LABEL

Patients express their awareness that death is inevitable in many ways and seek legitimization of their labeling themselves as dying from the people around them. As will become apparent, patients eventually learn their fates, whether or not they are told directly. In most instances they are not told by an explicit statement such as "you are going to die," but by the cues they receive from changes in the interactional processes going on around them. Some of the many ways patients expressed that they recognized that dying was inevitable and some of the responses that contributed to their recognition are described below.

PATIENTS' METHODS OF KNOWING, SHARING, AND ACCEPTING THE LABEL OF DYING

Patients directly and indirectly expressed their understanding of the situation to other interactors. They expressed their recognition indirectly through religious practices, by relating dreams, folklore, or in other symbolic ways such as by accounting for farewells to loved ones. They expressed their knowledge directly by telling of their fears and by freely talking about their dying and approaching deaths.

Religion and Religious Beliefs. As discussed in Chapter 5, one indicator that death is believed to be imminent is the increased references to religious beliefs by all interactors and the encouragement of patients by nurses and physicians to rely upon their faith. There is also greater use and visibility of religious items and symbols, such as Bibles, religious pictures, rosary beads, and votive candles. The latter were not allowed to be lighted because of fire safety regulations.

In many instances clergy visited more frequently and were welcomed by patients. Sometimes family members feared such visits would alarm the patients, especially when the patient did not attend religious services regularly.

Dreams. Sharing of dreams was another symbolic way of communicating with others. About 10% of the patients expressed their recognition of the imminence of death by relating their dreams to someone. Two subjects spontaneously told the nurse/researcher about the following dreams.

The first example was from a 28-year-old man who, early in his admission, stated, "I know I have lymphoma and I know I have approximately two years to live. Now you know that I know, we all know that I know, so let's get on with it." Later he added, "I'm going to beat this thing; the whole thing is like a bad dream." However, as his symptoms progressed he stopped saying, "Don't worry, I'll beat this thing." Shortly before he died the following exchange occurred. It was 8:00 a.m.; he was lying quietly in bed. He was very pale and weak. His wife and four-year-old son were at his bedside. After exchanging the usual amenities, the following conversation took place.

Nurse/Researcher:	Dan, do you wish to wash up now or wait until your wife leaves? (Her usual pattern was to visit until around 10:00 a.m.)
Wife:	I think he would enjoy a bath. I'll leave and come back later.
Dan:	Yes, and I would like a nap. (His wife left, but before leaving the little boy climbed up on the bed.)
Child:	I love you Daddy.
Dan:	I love you, too, son; you'll never know how much.

(The nurse/researcher walked out of the room to give them privacy. Dan was obviously worse, his wife knew it. She had asked earlier in the morning how the nurse thought he was. His wife said he looked worse. The nurse/researcher expressed agreement.)

Dan:	(to nurse/researcher) Are you my nurse today?
Nurse/Researcher:	Yes.
Dan:	I'm so tired.
Nurse/Researcher:	Yes, Dan, you do look tired.
Dan:	I couldn't sleep last night; well, I could sleep, but I woke up at 3:00 a.m. It was terrible!
Nurse/Researcher:	It was terrible to wake up?
Dan:	I had a terrible dream. It was so awful. I had a terrible dream. (A long silence.)
Nurse/Researcher:	A terrible dream that woke you up?
Dan:	I dreamed I was in a contest. I tried and tried, but I couldn't win. It was terrible, I tried and tried but I couldn't win.

The nurse/researcher's interpretation of his use of this dream to communicate his knowledge that death was imminent and inevitable was confirmed when he expressed his appreciation of "open" conversation.

Dan:	Open is different from facts. Open is humanness and warmth, people who care how you feel, people who talk

to you; like you, you're here listening to me about *my dream. . . . my life.* Do you think anyone would listen to you about your dreams at that other place?

Cheryl, a 40-year-old woman in the terminal stages of acute myelogenous leukemia, also expressed her recognition of her imminent death through relating a dream. She had been seriously ill previously and had undergone brain surgery. Cheryl began the conversation with the nurse by talking about that surgery and then went on to tell about the dream she had after the operation.

Cheryl: I dreamed I was walking through a garden full of beautiful flowers. They were all different colors and the sun was shining. The doctor told me that meant I would get well. I had a terrible dream last night. It was all dark, there was no sun shining. I guess that means the opposite.

Folklore. Other patients express their awareness of their dying through symbols in the form of folklore or family understandings. They describe seeing or talking to deceased family members and receiving invitations to join them.

Many families have personal ways for dying patients to disclose their awareness of dying without mentioning the words dying or death. The following excerpt describes one such incident which also involved Cheryl. The nurse/researcher thought Cheryl was going to tell her how ill she was when she said, "Last night I heard the birds at the window." She seemed perfectly coherent, yet this discussion about birds at the window seemed to make little sense. The nurse/researcher responded, "you heard birds at the window last night?" Cheryl smiled and took the nurse/researcher's hand but said no more. When the nurse/researcher left the room, Cheryl's sister, who had been standing in the corridor, asked what Cheryl had said. She was told about the "birds at the window."

Sister: (crying) Oh, she knows she is dying; we thought she did, but weren't sure. She knows she is dying.
Nurse/Researcher: How do you know?
Sister: In our family there is an old belief that when you are about to die you will hear birds at the window.

Farewells. Another way patients expressed their recognition that death was imminent was through their need to be sure that they had said farewells to loved ones. One patient's husband called the nurse/researcher from the bedside of another patient. He looked so upset the nurse/researcher thought his wife had died.

Husband: My wife wants you, she wants to talk to you *alone.* (He waited outside with the patient's brothers while the nurse/researcher went into the room.)
Nurse/Researcher: You wanted to talk to me, Carol?
Carol: Yes.

The nurse/researcher sat by her bed in silence. Carol reached for her hand. They sat hand-in-hand looking at each other for a moment.

Carol: Count them, did I say goodbye to all my brothers? I have
                            lost count and I wanted to say goodbye to them all.
They went over the names together until Carol was satisfied she had said
goodbye to them all. She then fell asleep. When the nurse/researcher went back
into the corridor, the family was waiting.

Brother 1:   What did she want, what did she say?

Nurse/Researcher: She said she wanted to be sure she said goodbye to all
                            her brothers.

The three brothers stood with tears streaming down their faces.

Brother 2:   We are here, she said goodbye to us.

These examples demonstrate how patients communicate their awareness
that dying is inevitable and death imminent. In addition, they illustrate that exchange of information between health care providers and other interactors may
result in consensus about the situation of the patient.

In Cheryl's case, the exchange between the nurse/researcher and Cheryl,
followed by the discussion with her sister, clarified the meaning of the "birds at
the window" for the researcher, and confirmed the sister's suspicion that Cheryl
recognized that she was dying. In Carol's case, the request to speak with the
nurse/researcher and the consequential sharing of information with the brothers
confirmed that each interactor interpreted the situation in a similar way.

In each of the instances, the patient expressed knowledge of the imminence
of death to the nurse/researcher, who was assumed to have understood the
message.* In general, these patients selected the person(s) in whom to confide,
and this was usually a non-family member. Although patients could have selected any interactor as a confidant, they frequently selected nurses, who spent
more time with patients than other health care providers. Dying patients and
family members often protected themselves and each other by not confronting
the issue of death directly. They revealed their knowledge about the situation to
and through a nurse, whom they apparently believed already knew that the patient was dying and therefore would not be upset if the issue were raised. Even in
those situations where families had personal ways to disclose their awareness
that dying was expected, the message frequently was communicated through the
nurse, as in the case of Cheryl. This triadic pattern of communication is discussed in more detail later in this chapter.

Fears. The expression of fears is another common method the patients used
to communicate knowledge that they were dying and would soon be dead. The
most frequently expressed fear was that of abandonment, especially by their physicians. Some of this fear of abandonment may have been stimulated by the fact
that as active medical therapy became less effective, physicians interacted with
patients less. They did not abandon their patients, but as there was less medical
therapy to oversee, their visiting patterns changed. Increasingly, the physicians

---

*It is important to note that body language, such as hand-holding, is interpreted as a
sign of understanding the other's view of the situation. Cheryl interpreted the nurse/
researcher's silence and hand-holding as confirmation that the meaning of "the birds at
the window" was jointly understood.

relied upon reports from nurses about the patient's condition, and expected nurses to provide the necessary comfort and emotional support to the patient and family. They usually were not present when a patient died but expected to be notified so that they could inform the family that the patient had died.

The patients who expressed fear of abandonment described changes in their physicians' behaviors which they interpreted as signs of abandonment or impending abandonment. Some patients said that their physicians visited as frequently as before but did not stay as long. Others expressed that their physicians visited less often. Still others complained that their physicians either did not answer their questions or did not stay long enough for them to ask questions. Some stated that their physicians just looked at them, nodded and left the room without speaking.

Many patients told nurses about their symptoms and complaints of discomfort, but refused to share these with their physicians even when encouraged to do so. A few patients stated that their physicians did not take their complaints seriously. Others interpreted their physicians' lack of verbal response to their physical complaints or questions as a form of disapproval. It was as though patients believed that they had not fulfilled their part of the bargain with their physicians. It was as if they feared that their physicians would continue to care for them only if they responded to treatment by getting well or at least by not getting sicker.

In addition to fearing abandonment, patients expressed other fears. They told of their concerns for their families and regrets for having to leave them.

Another frequently expressed fear was that of dying while asleep. The following conversation between Cheryl, who had described "hearing the birds at the window" (p. 82), and the nurse/researcher illustrates her fear of abandonment by her physician and by loved ones, as well as her need for a personal confidant who was not a family member.

It was 12:30 a.m., Cheryl had been crying on and off throughout the evening. When the nurse/researcher entered the room, Cheryl just looked at her. The nurse/researcher said, "What's the matter, Cheryl, can't you sleep?" Cheryl did not answer; she looked at the nurse/researcher as tears streamed down her cheeks. The nurse/researcher sat down beside her bed. Cheryl took her hand, and holding the nurse/researcher's pressed both their hands to the nurse/researcher's cheek and said "I like that." She was silent for a few moments and then she asked if the nurse/researcher read the Bible. The conversation then turned to her thoughts about her past experiences as a child in a large family. Just as abruptly she stated that she just could not sleep.

Nurse/Researcher: Why can't you sleep, Cheryl?
Cheryl: Oh, I don't know.
Nurse/Researcher: Have you ever had difficulties sleeping before?
Cheryl: No, not really.
Nurse/Researcher: Why do you suppose you are having difficulty sleeping tonight? (pause) Are you uncomfortable? (pause) Are you worried? (pause)

When she did not respond, the nurse/researcher said:
Cheryl, are you afraid to go to sleep?
Her eyes lit up and she said:
That's exactly it, I'm afraid to go to sleep.

Nurse/Researcher:	What makes you afraid to go to sleep?
Cheryl:	Oh, I don't know.
Nurse/Researcher:	Are you afraid you won't wake up?

Again her eyes brightened and she looked at the nurse/researcher.

Cheryl:	Yes, that's it, I'm afraid I'll never wake up again. My daughter, you know, is 17, and her boyfriend Peter was 18 and he just died in the hospital. He had leukemia like me. He just went to sleep and never woke up.
Nurse/Researcher:	Do you think that will happen to you?
Cheryl:	It might, it might happen to me. Do you think it will happen to me?
Nurse/Researcher:	I really don't know if that will ever happen to you, Cheryl, but I don't think it will happen tonight.
Cheryl:	Oh, I'm so glad. The only thing I want is to go home, to be with my family. I really want to go home. Do you think Dr. Z. will still take care of me?
Nurse/Researcher:	Do you think he won't?
Cheryl:	Oh, I think Dr. Z. will take care of me. He has always taken care of me. Do you think he will stick with me?
Nurse/Researcher:	Yes, Cheryl, I think Dr. Z. will stick with you. I don't think he will ever pull out on you. He will come in and see you and do everything he can to help you, just like he always has.
Cheryl:	Do you think he can cure me?
Nurse/Researcher:	No, I don't think he can cure you, but he has kept your leukemia in control before, perhaps he can keep it in control again.
Cheryl:	Yes, my leukemia is out of control. I really don't feel well. All I want to do is go home. You know, it's a wonderful thing that you will sit here and talk with me. All the girls [nursing staff] will come in and sit down and talk with me. It's a wonderful thing. It makes you feel people really care and you can always depend on the nurses to come and sit and talk with you.
	Everyone should have a wonderful husband like mine. My husband will always come, he will always be there. He comes all the time and he will come whenever I call and that's a wonderful thing, too. It's a wonderful thing to have all the people around you who are kind and nice.

(At this point she looked very sleepy and was obviously fighting to stay awake.)

Nurse/Researcher:	Would you like to sleep now, Cheryl?
Cheryl:	Not if you're going to leave.
Nurse/Researcher:	How about if I sit here while you close your eyes and see if you can't fall asleep? I'll tell the other nurses to look in on you when I leave.
Cheryl:	Oh, yes, I would like that. (She fell asleep in about 15 minutes.)

FAMILY MEMBERS' RECOGNITION, COMMUNICATIONS, AND VERIFICATIONS OF THE LABEL OF DYING

Family members as well as patients communicate their recognition of the *dying* label or request verification of their labeling the patient as the *dying patient*. Like the patients, family members communicate their initial labeling of the patient as *dying* through the expression of fears. These fears, however, are related to their own roles in the situation and in the future. Family members generally are concerned that they will not recognize the signs of imminent death. Most family members felt obligated to be present at the precise moment death occurred. Consequently, they pressed for predictions of the specific time of death. In addition, they frequently expressed concerns regarding their future without the dying person and regrets about past decisions or events.

Conversations regarding these subjects were usually with hospital personnel. In most instances, interactions containing the most provocative questions occurred in the corridors or in front of the elevators. Although family members were invited to "come and sit and talk in a more private place," they generally refused. It seemed as though they wanted explicit answers to their questions, but somehow asking them in a spontaneous, almost fleeting fashion made the answer less ominous. In fact, this pattern of interacting did allow the family member some control over the timing and duration of the interaction and the depth and amount of information they received. It also allowed them an escape route. They often terminated the interaction by walking away, by making a request, or asking an unrelated question.

Although these interactions were, or appeared to be, spontaneous, it was apparent that the decision to ask questions was not made hastily. In almost every instance, the questions were introduced by the comments, "I've been waiting for you," or "I've been thinking." Family members' need for a confidant or advisor is reflected in their selecting a specific nurse to talk to and requesting that they call each other by their first names. Family members generally preferred to ask questions of the nurses, at least initially, rather than directly seeking information from physicians.

There are many possible explanations for this behavior. Social distance between physicians and visitors is usually greater than it is between nurses and visitors. The information obtained from a nurse may seem less ominous than information coming from a physician who may be seen as having the final answer. There is also the more simple explanation of expediency; nurses are there at all times and thus are always immediately available.

The following is a representative illustration.

The patient was a 40-year-old man. His condition had grown progressively worse over the previous two weeks. His wife had been with him throughout this period. His pattern of living-dying was that of a three-step *descending plateau* (p. 70). The patient's wife approached the nurse/researcher in front of the elevators in the presence of many visitors. The visitors stepped back as the conversation began.

Wife:	Nurse, I've been waiting for you. How is my husband? I didn't want to talk in front of him.
Nurse/Researcher:	How does he look to you?

Wife:	Terrible! He looks terrible! What will I do when he is gone? I thought I would ask you, what will I do when he is gone? Do you think it will be tonight—should I stay?
Nurse/Researcher:	You look tired, Mrs. G., why don't you get some rest. You can stay if you like, but I don't think it will be necessary. Is there someone who can stay with you?
Wife:	My sister is with me. Will you talk with the doctor and tell me what he thinks?
Nurse/Researcher:	Would you like to talk with the doctor? He is here.
Wife:	No, you ask him about my husband and then tell me.
Nurse/Researcher:	Would you like me to come with you and you can talk with the doctor?
Wife:	No. I want *you* to talk with the doctor and then tell me what he says. *You* ask him about my husband.

As was true with the patients, the confirmation of the family members' definition of the patient as dying is not always direct or communicated verbally. Hand-holding and watching the facial expressions of health care providers serve the same purpose, whether the act is intentional or not. Refer once again to Cheryl. She had slept throughout the night with her family in constant attendance. Her pattern of living-dying continued to be that of *peaks and valleys*. The following morning she insisted upon getting out of bed and collapsed. The family ran from the room as the nurse's aide and the nurse/researcher carried her back to bed. She appeared dead, had no pulse or blood pressure. Her pupils were dilated and she was cyanotic. The nurse/researcher was about to listen for a heartbeat, when Cheryl spoke to the aide. About ten minutes passed before the nurse/researcher was able to leave the room to speak to her family who were waiting in the hallway. Cheryl's sister spoke first:

Sister:	When I saw the look on your face, I knew she was bad.
Nurse/Researcher:	She's okay now.
Sister:	You really care what happens to her, I could tell by the look on your face.

NURSES AND PHYSICIANS: INFORMATION EXCHANGE AND LABEL CONFIRMATION

Nurses and physicians, no less than other interactors, exchanged information to confirm their own labeling of a patient as *dying* and to evaluate the patient's recognition of his own dying status. Their observations were shared in face-to-face interactions and through written records, such as physicians' progress notes and nursing notes.

How, and if, this information was shared was dependent upon the physician's philosophy. Although internists were more apt than surgeons to share prognostic predictions directly and openly with nurses and family members, there was great variation among physicians of both groups. Patients usually were not directly told that death was unavoidable and imminent.

The following comments, written on the same day about the same patient, show one way of confirming the label. The first is a nurse's note, the second an excerpt from a physician's progress note.

Nurses's Note

Continues to ooze dark liquid guiac positive stool. Rectum tender to touch. Ate dry cereal at breakfast. States he is afraid to eat for fear of increasing his diarrhea. Patient depressed and wishes to die.

Physician's Note

See nurse's notes: The situation is as she describes. He is resigned to his fate, the family recognizes the situation. He is not in respiratory distress and he is very poor.

Another way the label is confirmed is through a code known to hospital personnel. Most hospitals use a code name when a patient requires cardiopulmonary resuscitation (CPR). This hospital was no exception. A "code three" (not the term used in this hospital) referred to a medical emergency needing immediate attention and a supreme effort to save the life of a patient whose respirations or heartbeat had stopped. It included using all known therapies, mechanical equipment, and extraordinary means necessary to maintain life through a temporary crisis period. When it was decided that CPR would be inappropriate and at best would serve only to prolong dying unnecessarily, the patient was designated a "no code three."

The decision as to whether a patient was a "no code three" was usually made by the physician in conjunction with the responsible family member(s). Nurses frequently asked physicians if a patient was a "no code three" or pressed them for a definitive decision.

The decision about what means were to be taken was necessary for nurses since they would be the ones who would initiate the call for a "code three" and would be responsible for beginning CPR measures. The knowledge was also functional in terms of interactions with patients and family members who, as described, frequently requested information from nurses regarding the dying label.

The following are some comments made by nurses and nursing personnel regarding the meaning and use of the "no code three." The information sought from each respondent was: (1) What does a "no code three" mean? (2) Does it make a difference in your care? and (3) How does it make a difference?

Conversation with a Licensed Practical Nurse (LPN).

LPN: A "no code three" means that if a patient dies you don't try to bring him back.

Nurse/Researcher: What do you mean, "bring him back?"

LPN: You know, you don't pound on his chest or do cardiac massage. It means there is nothing you can do.

Nurse/Researcher: Does that mean you don't take care of them?

LPN: No. It means you keep them comfortable and do their treatments and stuff. You call a doctor and everything like that.

Nurse/Researcher: Were you ever there when a patient with a "no code three" died?

LPN: Yes, one time I was but an RN was there, too.

Nurse/Researcher: What happened?

LPN: The RN called the house doctor and they did IV's

	[intravenous] and things but they didn't call a "code three."
Nurse/Researcher:	What happens when you call a "code three?"
LPN:	The whole team comes and you get the emergency cart.

Another example involving a Registered Nurse (RN):

Nurse/Researcher:	What does a "no code three" mean?
RN:	It means you do everything except cardiopulmonary resuscitation.
Nurse/Researcher:	If you know a person is a "no code three," does it make a difference in your care?
RN:	Sure, it's good to know if a patient is a "no code three" because then you know what to do.
Nurse/Researcher:	What do you mean by "what to do?"
RN:	Well, if a patient is a "no code three" then you know you can talk to the family better and then you can answer the patient's questions better.
Nurse/Researcher:	What kinds of questions?
RN:	Well, they (the family) ask you when the patient will die. Even if you don't know when they will die, at least you can be honest about the fact that they are dying and it will be soon. That way, the family can get the information they want, and lots of times you can start talking more freely with the patient.
Nurse/Researcher:	Does it help you care for the patient?
RN:	Yes, I think so because lots of times the patients say they want to die in peace and don't want machines and stuff and you can say that you won't use machines and things.

Physicians and nurses were conservative in their designation of a patient as a "no code three." Although at times its use served to legitimize the *dying* label, it more often served to alert interactors to the probable transition of the patient from the status of the *high risk of dying* to that of *dying patient*.

Thus far, examples have been provided as to how various types of interactors communicated their labeling or perception of the patient as the dying patient. The next question in the study explored the pathways of communication which led to common awareness and consequential labeling of the patient as dying by all interactors.

PATHWAYS OF COMMUNICATION

As demonstrated by earlier examples, the three types of interactors—patients, family members, and health care practitioners, including physicians, nurses, and nursing personnel—do not always communicate directly with each other. A triadic pattern of communication, or a series of triadic patterns, was identified where one type of interactor became an intermediary between the other two. In some instances, the family served as an intermediary between the health care providers and the patient. When this pattern occurred, the patient communicated directly with a family member who, in turn, transmitted the information to health care providers.

For instance, one patient never spoke of her dying to health care providers; in fact, her usual discussion with them concerned plans for future activities. However, she had asked her daughter to make formal plans for her funeral and she had selected her clothes, casket, and place of burial. The daughter provided the health care providers with this information.

More frequently, patients discussed their dying with health care providers, and family members discussed patients' dying with health care providers but not directly with each other. This pattern prevailed even when patients and family members were told of each other's views and concerns and were encouraged to talk together. Generally, the person who became the intermediary was able, or was perceived as being able, to view the situation from the perspective of the other interactors, regardless of whether the other interactors viewed the situation in the same way.

The intermediary served as a facilitator or as a blocking agent in the establishment of a definition of the situation common to all and in labeling the patient as the *dying patient.* Whether the intermediary served as a facilitator or a blocking agent depended upon the type of information they did or did not share with the other interactors and the understandings that developed about the further dissemination of this information.

Consistency in definitions and agreement on the label usually led to more frequent interactions on the part of all interactors, except when this agreement was premature in terms of the patient's time of biological death. The accomplishment of the labeling generally ends the indeterminancy of the situation. The labels give structure to the situation by giving each interactor a social identity. All interactors now have more specific labels and related roles, that is, the patient is the *dying patient,* the family is the family of the *dying patient.* Having commonly defined the situation in terms of achieving consensus on the label, the interactors, especially the patient and family members, search for ways to adapt to the label.

PATTERNS OF ADAPTATION TO THE DYING LABEL

Although there are variations in the reactions of the patients and family members to the label, *the dying patient,* five analytically distinguishable patterns of adaptation emerged from the data. *Relief from uncertainty* and *escape* emerged from the patients' perspective; *permission to die, invitation to die,* and *relabeling as non-person* arose from the perspective of families. These patterns are called *patterns of adaptation* rather than *patterns of acceptance or adjustment* because a sense of yielding or giving in to the demands of the situation is inherent in each. The goal of each pattern is to restore some sense of harmony to a situation which is perceived as unalterable.

Adaptation to the label included adjusting to or becoming reconciled to the label and, thus, to the situation. The label is accepted in that it is agreed upon and is believed to be accurate. Adapting to the label does not reflect a value orientation toward dying. Neither does it reflect approval or disapproval of the label, or acceptance of dying as a favorable or unfavorable state of being.

The patterns evolved from the perspectives of the dying patients and their family members. Physicians, nurses, and other nursing personnel reacted to and acted upon the content of these patterns in defining the situation and in their responses to family and patients. Although these health care providers discussed the content with each other, they usually did not directly discuss the content with patients or family members. Two unwritten codes seem to guide behavior: (1) build upon the patients' and families' strengths; and (2) do not create any more conflict than already exists or is absolutely necessary.

The patterns of adaptation were not unique to any particular sex, socioeconomic, ethnic, or religious group. Religious beliefs influenced how, not if, the information was communicated and served as a means of endorsing behavior. Religiously oriented persons, regardless of denomination, more frequently used symbolic language such as "join God" or "go to heaven" than non-religiously oriented persons. In contrast, non-religiously oriented persons were generally more direct and more frequently used the words die, death, and dying than religiously oriented people.

In describing the patterns of adaptation of patients and families, reference will be made to the patterns of living-dying. There is no cause-effect relationship intended. These patterns of adaptation are neither mutually exclusive, nor is any one pattern of adaptation necessarily related to a particular living-dying pattern. There may or may not be a transition from one pattern to another. These patterns of adaptation exist as do the patterns of living-dying. Further empirical study is needed to link them in any definitive fashion.

PATIENTS' ADAPTATION PATTERNS

Two patterns of adaptation, *relief from uncertainty* and *escape*, evolved primarily from the perspective of dying patients. Other interactors, especially family members, sometimes expressed similar comments, but these were about dying patients or in response to the comments initiated by dying patients.

Relief from Uncertainty. The first pattern, relief from uncertainty, was characterized by searching for some form of closure by dealing with fate or the supernatural. Religiously oriented persons placed their future in the hands of a supernatural being, "It is up to God," "God's will be done." People who were not religiously oriented also relinquished responsibility for or control over any final decisions or judgments. They made such comments as "I'll just have to wait and see," or "I'll take it one step at a time."

Both religious and non-religious people recognized the limitations of modern medicine.

Religiously oriented people relied upon their belief in God's intervention. They made statements such as "God will help," "I believe in miracles." One 50-year-old woman who had undergone many surgeries for cancer and had recently completed a third course of chemotherapy stated: "I've been through enough suffering, but what happens now is up to God. He will give me time."

Non-religiously oriented people looked to the prior successes of modern science and medicine. One patient outlined the progress that had been made over the years in curing tuberculosis. Another discussed the critical nature of his health situation and the lack of known treatment, then added, "but something new is always being discovered." A third acknowledged that he was dying, but said, "There is always hope. The scientists may be working on something right now."

The relief from uncertainty pattern of adaptation was most apparent among people living and dying in a *peaks and valleys pattern*. Religious and non-religious patients had hope, yet at the same time yearned for closure. They wished for life or for death. There was an overriding "live while you live or die and be done with it" attitude.

The following excerpts illustrate the relief from uncertainty pattern of adaptation.

One patient, Mrs. L., made arrangements to see a faith healer. Mrs. L. was a pleasant person, the mother of three children. She was Protestant and described herself as "very religious." She had been diagnosed with metastatic lympho-epithelioma one year prior to her first admission to the medical center. She had been hospitalized on multiple occasions for radiation and chemotherapy.

She was nearly blind due to an inoperable tumor behind her eyes. Her dark brown eyes stared from her thin, very pale, skeletal face. Her spindle-like arms and bony shoulders looked misplaced above her grossly distended abdomen and edematous legs and feet.

Despite her suffering, she was concerned about her appearance. As she put it "just look at my hair [she was nearly bald from her chemotherapy], I must look a sight!" Her concern about her appearance was a reflection of her concern about her family. She was vehement about trying to hide her pain and suffering from them.

Pain and discomfort had become a part of her life and more and more were dominating her life. She had metastases to her bones and liver. Extensive ascites contributed to a paralytic ileus and to difficulty in breathing and moving about. Her treatment focused upon control of her pain and discomfort. Treating her ascites was essential. Thus, she was weighed every other day, a painful procedure for her.

Throughout her illness she stated that as long as she could walk, she knew she had time left. On the 56th day of this, her last hospital admission, she insisted that she be discharged. She refused to give any explanation and remained sullen and thoughtful throughout the morning. She avoided any conversation with the nurse/researcher and other interactors.

The following conversation took place, as the nurse/researcher and another nurse were lifting her onto a scale to be weighed. Although it was usual for patients to express their fears and most troubling thoughts when nursing procedures were being done, the conversation came as a surprise to both nurses.

Patient:	I have to get out of here tomorrow, I have an appointment.
Nurse:	(surprised) You do?
Patient:	Yes, I have an important appointment. (The nurse continued to weigh her and she said) Wait, rub my feet, they are numb. (While the nurse was rubbing her feet, the patient looked at the nurse/researcher and in rapid succession questioned.) I'm never going to walk again,

	am I? Can you get me a wheelchair to take home with me? I have a very important appointment.
Nurse/Researcher:	What is this appointment?
Patient:	Well, I have to go Friday to talk with (name of faith healer). I went there before to watch. There was a 13-year-old who never walked, now she can. She cured her. (There were tears in her eyes as she reached up for the nurse/researcher's hand. They held hands for a moment.) I'm going Friday, it took me a long time to get an appointment. I believe in miracles, you don't believe in miracles. (There was a long pause.) Do you believe in miracles?
Nurse/Researcher:	Sometimes. (The nurse/researcher thought it was somewhat of a miracle that she was alive.)
Patient:	Well, I do. Miracles happen and I have to go on Friday.

Although the arrangements were made to take Mrs. L. to see the faith healer, she never did see her. Mrs. L. lost consciousness on Thursday night and died two days later.

Another example is that of Mrs. D.S., a 70-year-old Roman Catholic with acute granulocytic leukemia. Mrs. D.S. was a gentle, soft-spoken, attractive little woman, who spoke English well although she was born in Italy. She lived with and cared for her 80-year-old husband.

She, like Mrs. L., had multiple admissions to the hospital for chemotherapy and for the complications of her disease. Mrs. D.S. was routinely admitted for two days every three weeks to receive blood transfusions.

Customarily she greeted the nurse/researcher with a hug and a kiss on the cheek, but her admission on the night of September 7 was different. She had begun to bleed internally. She spoke of her fears of not being able to care for herself and of becoming a burden to her children. She wept as she spoke of her temporary living arrangement: one week with each child.

She remorsefully stated, "You know I was here, very sick, I was bleeding in my stomach, they saved me. I don't know what they saved me for; now I have to wait for it to happen again, it would have been better to die than be like this, waiting." Mrs. D.S. recovered from this episode, returned to her husband and their apartment, and resumed living.

She was readmitted to the hospital on October 30 with more symptoms of bleeding. She was extremely frightened, and grabbed the nurse/researcher's hand and refused to release it even while the physician examined her. When the physician left the room, Mrs. D.S. lay very quietly, still holding the nurse/researcher's hand, looked up and said: "I told you last time, they shouldn't have done anything, now I have to go through it all again."

She was to return home for a short time only to be readmitted with hepatitis. Her appearance and behavior were changed. She was extremely frail, thin, and had dark circles around her eyes, which were no longer bright and sparkling. She still smiled when the nurse/researcher entered the room, reached for her hand and kissed it. She looked directly into the nurse/researcher's eyes and said, "I'm not any better." The nurse/researcher responded: "Yes, I know." Mrs. D.S.'s eyes filled with tears for a moment. Then she went to sleep. Once again she returned home. Her parting words to the nurse/researcher were, "I'm going home now, they couldn't make me better, maybe I'll be back, maybe not, God bless you."

Mrs. D.S. had a total of 27 admissions during a two-year period. She died in the hospital on December 15, but before she did she said:

> I hope I die soon. I told you last time, they shouldn't have done anything, now I have to go through it again. I think I'm dying. I know I'm dying, don't you think I'm dying? Pray for me, pray that I die without any pain. [She reached over and kissed the nurse/researcher's fingers and touched her own forehead. The nurse/researcher brushed her lips against her forehead. Mrs. D.S. smiled and said] Don't forget, you said you would pray for me. [The nurse/researcher nodded, yes. The patient turned and said] God bless you, God bless you, remember me.

Other patients with histories similar to Mrs. D.S. made similar statements. One woman said:

> These doctors aren't doing a thing for me! I'm miserable and fed up with things. I look a mess, my hair is falling out again. I wish it would either end or I'll get all better. It's all up to God now. I pray, "please God, take me."

A man in his thirties described his course by saying:

> It's just up and down, up and down. It seems like it will never end. There isn't too much left to try [the reference was to further treatment]. Maybe they'll discover something. I wish one way or another it would end.

Still another patient, a 48-year-old woman who had metastatic cancer and had been admitted to the hospital on multiple occasions for treatment, stated: "I've been through enough suffering, but what happens now is up to God. He will give me time."

Escape. The second pattern of adaptation, *escape*, was characterized by: (1) resignation, and (2) escape from loneliness and despair. This pattern of adaptation frequently appeared among patients with the *gradual slant* pattern of living-dying.

The following are examples of the circumstances under which this pattern evolved and the comments of patients.

Mrs. G. was an 80-year-old woman with congestive heart failure. She was alert and active when first admitted to the hospital on September 18. She was very anxious and lonely. Much of her conversation focused upon her many somatic complaints which included chest pain, difficulty breathing, episodic mental confusion, gastrointestinal difficulties, and multiple aches and pains.

She had few visitors, received little mail, and a rare telephone call. She believed people did not take her symptoms very seriously. Her interpretation seemed accurate. Her death on September 24 took everyone by surprise.

She frequently stated: "I have nothing left to live for. I pray I die. I pray to God I die before I get put away in some home or other."

Another elderly patient, a 79-year-old widower with diabetes and congestive heart failure stated:

Dying is just another experience. I'm not afraid of dying. It can't be worse than lying here day after day, all alone with only nurses who care. No family, even my friends don't come any more.

FAMILY PATTERNS OF ADAPTATION

Permission to die, invitation to die, and *relabeling* the dying person as *non-person* were patterns of adaptation initiated by family members or significant others. The permission to die and invitation to die patterns will be discussed first since they are similar.

Permission to Die. The *permission to die* pattern of adapting was characterized by offering dying people consolation or granting them permission to die. The comments were usually initiated by a family member who had a close relationship with the dying person. The patient's living-dying pattern was frequently the *downward slope.* Although in many instances the patients had illnesses of a short duration which rapidly culminated in death, the provoking factors seemed to be the unremitting symptoms and suffering of the patient with no hope for recovery.

For example: Steve, a 14-year-old Roman Catholic, was well until September 10 when he developed abdominal pain. Four days later surgery was performed and a ruptured Meckel's diverticulum was discovered. Following surgery he developed D.I.C. (disseminated intravascular coagulation) and was transferred to the medical center. He had a stormy downhill course, which included seizures, sepsis, respiratory and cardiac arrests, more surgery, the use of respirators, cardiac monitors, renal dialysis, and multiple transfusions.

On admission to the medical center Steve was labeled *high risk of dying.* He was admitted to the surgical intensive care unit. His parents stayed at his bedside most of the time. Although he was unconscious, his parents talked to him. "We're here, Steve, we're here. Open your eyes, Steve, just try."

As Steve's condition worsened, his family searched for signs of improvement. They asked the nurses, "Has he opened his eyes at all? Do you think he hears us? Are the seizures less?" The nurses responded "no" to these questions.

His parents continued to encourage him "to try," "you will get better if you just try." His condition grew more grave and the family was informed that his recovery was not likely.

As the family members became more resigned to the fact that death was imminent and recovery not possible, the focus of their conversations changed. They made reference to life after death and sanctioned Steve's dying by granting him permission to stop trying to live.

His mother said: "It's okay [for you to die], we know you won't be apart from us; you pray for us when you're up there." His dad added, "It's okay, son, I'm getting old myself, and I'll be coming to join you, so you won't be alone."

The work ethic was operative for all in evaluating the situation of the dying person. Health care providers and other interactors condoned dying by referring to the patient's past performance. For instance, one woman turned to her husband and said:

You were a good husband, you always took good care of us. You tried, there's nothing more you can do. We understand.

Invitation to Die. The fourth pattern was the overt *invitation to die.* This pattern occurred in situations where the patient had been debilitated for a long period, usually months, with unrelenting pain and other discomfort. It was preceded by the evaluation that there was no further hope of recovery, that all available known treatments had been found ineffective, and that there had been a concerted effort on the part of the dying person to get well. In all instances where there was a direct invitation to die made to the patient, there had been *close* family relationships. Family members had actively and directly participated in caring for the patient, both in their homes and during hospital stays. In addition, members of the family or close friends were consistently present day, evening, and throughout the night while the patient was hospitalized. Usually, the patients had been involved in decisions regarding their treatments and activities throughout their illnesses for as long as they were able. In most instances, their invitation was made directly by a family member, but sometimes it was made through an intermediary, as was the case in the following example.

Mrs. G. was a 48-year-old woman with squamous cell carcinoma of the lung with metastasis. She was an attractive woman, appearing younger than her stated age, despite the fact that there was a large (7 cm in diameter), red and angry appearing lesion on the left side of her head. Her pattern of *living-dying* had been that of *peaks and valleys.* She had multiple courses and types of therapies including surgery, radiation, and chemotherapy. Her family and friends lauded her "tremendous will to live."

She and her family were practicing Roman Catholics. They were active in their church and relied upon their faith for comfort. Mrs. G. repeatedly made reference to the "will of God." Members of the clergy visited her regularly.

She and her husband were happily married. They frequently spoke of the joys they shared together. They had no children. Because they both enjoyed their time together, Mrs. G. frequently refused her medication for pain and Mr. G. requested that she receive her medication at a time which would not make her so sleepy during their visits. They both looked forward to celebrating their 20th anniversary on January 14.

The following conversation took place on December 21, in the corridor outside Mrs. G.'s room. A close friend of the patient stopped the nurse/researcher as she left Mrs. G.'s room.

Friend:	I don't know how you do it. You are all so patient with George [the patient's husband] even when he won't let you give pain medication. I told him to stop thinking about himself and think of her and her pain. He just thinks about himself, you know?
Nurse/Researcher:	He loves her very much and wants to keep her as long as he can. We do medicate her about every four hours. We worry about him too, but this is perhaps more difficult for him than it is for her right now.
Friend:	I think you are right. He knows she is going to die, we told him to tell her to give up, that it is *enough* already; he *won't* do it.
Mother:	[Name of clergyman] has been in to see her. He said he

told her that it was time to stop fighting, that she had fought hard and long enough. She should rest now and let God's will be done. She has done her best and we are proud of her, but she should stop fighting and join God in Heaven.

A few days later her husband made the following comment to the nurse/researcher:

She has always had such a strong will to live and has always been such a fighter, but now I pray she will stop fighting and go to sleep in peace. She has suffered enough, you can't make her better. I shall have to tell her it is time to join God.

Mrs. G. died on January 4.

Another example of the *invitation to die* involved a mother and her 28-year-old son, Jeff. Jeff had been treated for Hodgkin's disease over a period of three years. He was essentially well until the last month of his illness when he progressed to stage 4B and developed pulmonary infiltrates and sepsis. Medical treatments were ineffective. He was extremely restless and uncomfortable. His mother looked at him as though she were talking to an overtired, obstreperous, but much loved child who needed a nap, and simply and directly stated: "Jeff, Jeff darling, why don't you just die?"

Of interest is the belief that just as patients can be instrumental in recovering and are expected *to try*, they can also be instrumental in dying and thus, they are relinquished from their responsibility of *trying* in the form of *permission to die* or *an invitation to die*. They are, in fact, then expected to comply and to die. This phenomenon will be discussed further, along with the role of the dying patient.

Relabel as Non-Person. The last pattern of adaptation evolved in situations where the dying patient was no longer perceived as a person, especially by family members. It occurred predominantly in situations where: (1) the patient was no longer able to communicate in some interpretable and therefore meaningful way, either verbally or non-verbally; (2) this non-communicative state was persistent and consistent; and (3) it did not culminate in death within some predictable time period, but death was seen as inevitable. It differs from the other patterns in that the interactions were usually between family members and health care providers only.

More succinctly stated, the process was ended when the patient could no longer interact. This occurred when the patient no longer displayed a social self or interpreted the actions of others. The patient was dead and life was ended.

However, the patient was not biologically dead. Therein lay the dilemma. W. I. Thomas' dictum "If men define situations as real, they are real in their consequences" may be so, but only to a degree. The patient was biologically alive, although perceived as dead, socially at least. This perception influenced interactions, but did not change the fact that the patient was biologically alive.

The following emotionally charged comments made to the nurse/researcher reflected the dilemma.

The patient was a 35-year-old businessman with lymphosarcoma. He was married and had three small children. His wife had been active in caring for him. She was instrumental in making it possible for him to die at home.

Patient's Wife: I've had it, I just can't take it any more. He's unconscious, he just lies there. That's not him. It's a terrible thing, I just can't stand to look at him any more. It's terrible, that Kubler-Ross makes it sound easy. Well, she surely over-simplified things. I never knew it was going to be any-thing like this. . . . She doesn't tell you anything about the way it's really going to be.

Patient's Mother: I've done my crying now. I just want him peaceful. He can't do anything. He can't be anything, he can't even talk anymore. When you can't talk you are not a person. What are you people doing anyway? Can't you do something to end all this?

THE DYING LABEL: EVOLUTION AND CONSEQUENCES

In the same way that patients are not simultaneously labeled as the *dying patient* by all interactors at any one identifiable time, they do not assume nor are they accorded all the rights and obligations that accompany this label at any one definitive time. There is convergence when most interactors label the patient as the *dying patient* and when death is predicted within a matter of hours. The label, *the dying patient*, is not fixed or stable. It arises as people make inferences about the behaviors of the individuals around them. These inferences lead to more inferences and the consequential fluctuation of the label.

As patients become labeled as *dying patients*, they and their families are accorded different rights and obligations. The assumption of these obligations and the giving of these rights provide further cues which both legitimize the label and contribute to achieving consensus about the situation by other interactors who did not recognize the progression of the patient from *high risk of dying* to *dying*. But even as the label is being confirmed by interactors, it is continually being negated, for labeling itself is a dialectical process.

The label, the *dying patient*, is accompanied by rights and privileges not ac-corded to patients who are expected to get well or not expected to die within a predicted period of time, especially not during the present hospital admission. For instance, patients labeled as *high risk of dying* but bordering on the dying patient end of the continuum are allowed and encouraged to express emotions such as anger or depression. Visiting hours become more relaxed. Special re-quests for changes in the scheduling of treatments and for favorite foods are honored. These patients are expected, nonetheless, to comply with modifications of medical treatments and are encouraged and expected to "try" to get well. Such decisions are not formal, nor are they made by any one person. They arise as interactors act and react to each other's behaviors. Although the label *dying pa-tient* is not necessarily permanent, it does have consequences.

As the label is accepted or confirmed by more interactors and as death is seen as inevitable and discharge from the hospital unlikely, rules related to get-ting well are further relaxed and rules related to dying are adopted. Since health care providers are more able to predict the hour of death, they institute a more rapid transition from the use of rules for *high risk of dying* to the use of rules for *dying patients*.

For instance, visiting hours are completely relaxed. Family members are not only encouraged but are expected to visit the patient. Arrangements are made for visitors to sleep in the patient's room and to join the patient at meal times if they desire. Family members who do not visit regularly, or who are judged as not interested or not supportive of the dying patient, are seen in a negative light by other patients, visitors, and health care providers. These family members are made aware of the expectation that they be there by such comments as, "Your husband was calling for you for hours," and, "Oh, it's so good you could come; that will make her so much happier."

Therapeutic regimes are discontinued or ignored. Dying patients are allowed to decide whether or not they want to take their medications, eat their meals, or get out of bed. In other words, they do not have to try to get well.

The dying patient is entitled to make demands that disrupt the normal routine of other interactors. Family members change their daily work schedules, babysitters care for children, hospital routines are ignored or are adapted to meet the patient's requests. The patients and also their family members are entitled to be impolite and to make greater demands upon the time of health care providers.

Once the patient has been labeled as *dying* and a supreme effort is made by health care providers and family members to grant privileges, the patient is expected to die within the predicted period of time. Patients who do not die but whose physical conditions improve are relabeled as *high risk of dying* and they resume the rights and obligations of that label. If patients do not die when expected, and there is no improvement in their physical condition, they remain labeled as the *dying patient*; however, the rights accompanying this label are gradually taken away. Interactors are expected to make sacrifices in terms of their own life-styles for only a defined period of time. If death does not occur within two weeks or, at most, a month following the predicted date of death, especially if the patient has been relabeled as non-person, family members withdraw and are encouraged to withdraw and return to their former patterns of living. Under these conditions patients have few visitors and frequently die alone or only with nurses or other nursing personnel present.

When it is accepted by most interactors that the patient will die within an expected, predicted period of time, their care becomes primarily the responsibility of nursing staff. Physicians are expected to visit and communicate with nurses, but the responsibility for continued interactions with family members and patients is delegated to and accepted by nurses. This agreement is evident in the following statement made by a physician to a nurse, regarding a patient who was expected to die within a few days.

> There is nothing we can do; that thing [cancer] has attacked everything— lungs, spleen, everything. [He turned to the nurse.] Go and help them [family and patient], go talk to them. You're her nurse today, you go talk to them. You should be able to help them; I've done all I can.

Identifiable rights and obligations develop with the label and, in turn, serve to confirm the label. Labeling is functional in structuring the situation and establishing a division of labor. There are dysfunctional consequences, however, when the patient is prematurely labeled as the *dying patient*.

As stated previously, there were rights and obligations which accompanied this label. One obligation was to die as expected. People were sanctioned for not dying when expected. These sanctions took the form of withdrawal on the part of other interactors. Thus, premature labeling could result in isolating dying people from significant others. It also could cause them to be treated as non-persons, thus creating a social death while they were biologically very much alive.

SUMMARY

Two different social labels were identified in this study: namely, *high risk of dying* and the *dying patient*. The label of *high risk of dying*, based upon diagnosis, prognosis, and course of illness, offered greater structure than the *dying patient* label. Patients became labeled the *dying patient* when there was common agreement that death was inevitable within a predictable period of time. This common agreement and its consequential labeling evolved through interactions and sharing of information. There was no one well-defined place in time when the person was initially labeled as *dying* by all interactors.

Patients communicated their knowledge of the imminence of their own death directly and indirectly. Indirect means included increased emphasis on religious faith, use of dreams and other symbolic means to express feelings, and the expression of fears such as abandonment or dying in their sleep.

Family members also communicated their recognition of the patient's imminent death and their labeling of the patient as *dying* through the expression of fears. Their fears were related to their present and future roles with the patient and their concern over being able to recognize the signs of impending death so that they could fulfill their felt obligation to be present at the time of actual death.

Health care providers communicated their views about how a patient should be labeled in face-to-face interactions with each other and through their written records. They also used a coded language to assist in defining the situation and labeling the patient.

There was a triadic pattern of communication with different interactors serving as the intermediary at different times and for differing reasons. Through the use of triadic patterns of communication, the definition of the situation was revised or reinforced and resulted in changing the label from the *high risk of dying patient* to that of the *dying patient*. The latter label ended the indeterminancy of the situation, which led the interactors to adopt differing patterns of adaptation. There were five patterns of adaptation. The two that evolved from the perspective of the patient were *relief from uncertainty* and *escape*. The other patterns, described as *permission to die*, *invitation to die*, and *relabel as non-persons*, were initiated by family members and significant others.

Labels were neither fixed nor stable. They both influenced and were influenced by the behavior of interactors. Labels were accompanied by certain rights and obligations with the rights and obligations changing as the label changed.

7   Identities, Roles, Negotiations, and Consensus

THE HOSPITAL AND NEGOTIATIONS FOR ORDER

T he hospital is a place where there is a continual negotiation for order. There is pressure to achieve consensus about the situation and how people are to act in the situation even as other interactors—health care providers, patients, and others—are directing their activities toward cure or maintenance of optimal patient function. The situation of and surrounding dying persons differs only in degree from that of patients who are acutely or chronically ill.

The process of negotiation is the same for all interactors in the situation. Each interactor has an interpretation or opinion about the situation. When interactors discover that their opinions contradict, conflict, or are incongruent with the opinions of others in the social environment, there is an exchange of views. Each interactor influences the other; opinions are modified to reach mutual agreement or consensus about the situation.

Negotiations for mutual agreements or consensus about the situation of and surrounding dying patients are not only more apparent, but also are more essential than in the situation of acutely and chronically ill patients. Because there is little structure in the situation of the dying patient, there is a continual searching for structure, bargaining for rules of behavior, and negotiating for identities and roles. Agreements are reached, revised, and discarded and, in some cases, ignored or forgotten, at the same time as they continually are being established, renewed, and reviewed. Negotiations lead to further negotiations. Agreements from the various negotiating processes do not occur by chance but are patterned in terms of who contacted whom, when, for what reasons, and under what conditions. In addition, there are agreements as to how long a particular understanding will remain in effect.

The agreements, whether related to the label of dying, the identities or roles of patients, interactors, or rules of behavior, constitute common definitions of the situation that are always subject to revision as the interactional conditions fluctuate and as patients' physical conditions change.

This chapter explores how common definitions of the situations evolved, and identifies the processes and factors that contributed to role formation of the interactors, such as the rules for behavior and the process of negotiation. The rules governing and influencing behavior are discussed first.

RULES FOR BEHAVIOR

NORMS

There are generally no formal or binding rules concerning the behavior of any interactors which are not negotiable. The situation is not, however, completely amorphous. The negotiating process occurs within the confines of state laws and professional and societal conventions. Although the norms provide guidelines as to the range of behavior appropriate and applicable to the care of acutely and chronically ill patients, they are not so useful in guiding interactions with and regarding dying patients.

Most interactors were aware of multiple and potentially incongruent norms about dying patients. The recognition of conflicting norms by the interactors contributed to their inability to accept one norm as superior to another. The inability of interactors to choose one norm over another often resulted in their withdrawal from the situation or their refusal to commit themselves to any norm or set of norms.

For example, a patient requests that treatment be discontinued and that life not be prolonged artificially, but the patient also asks to remain in a hospital directed toward cure. Does complying with a patient's request that available treatment not be used constitute a form of passive euthanasia which violates the norm regarding bodily harm to patients? Or does continuance of treatment against a patient's wishes constitute a form of harm to a patient since the patient is denied the right to die with dignity? What are the legal and moral implications and consequences of either choice?

Of interest in this regard was the introduction of a "living will" by two patients in the study. They signed documents requesting that no "heroic" measures or extraordinary means be employed to prolong living and that they be allowed to die with dignity under such conditions as no probable return to productive living, intractable pain, or agony. There are many issues related to "living wills." First, definitions are problematic. Who determines what constitutes heroic measures? What is productive living? What constitutes dying with dignity? Secondly, the "living will" was not a legally binding document at the time data were collected. Whether or not it was honored depended upon all the interactors and the surrounding conditions. The "living will" is important since it provides an example of the patient's involvement in negotiating for agreements and understandings. More importantly, it reflects the impact of social movements, in this instance consumer input, on decisions made by the hospital representatives and workers.

The patients who signed the "living wills" both died in the hospital. One patient died while receiving multiple forms of aggressive therapy. The other patient died shortly after therapy was discontinued.

Decisions were made as various factors were weighed. Patients had to be cared for, so health care professionals had to act. There were rules of behavior related to the care of patients in general and the dying patient in particular. The rules are best described as agreements and understandings. Although most interactors distinguished between agreements and understandings, they did not use the terms. Since there was a relationship between the agreements and understandings and the process of negotiation, they will be described before discussing negotiations per se.

AGREEMENTS AND UNDERSTANDINGS

Agreements and understandings differed in terms of duration. *Agreements* were long-standing arrangements between and among all interactors in the situation. In many instances the agreements existed prior to the entrance of the observed interactors. In these situations, they emanated both from the greater society and from within the hospital and were easily identified and generally known by all in the situation. Nonetheless, they were presented in "for instance" terms with comparison to analogous incidents, not as universals. They were generally honored since they provided some structure to the situation by serving as a kind of starting point or frame of reference, especially in regard to the division of labor.

The following is an example of such an *agreement*. All interactors accepted that private physicians had the right and responsibility to inform the patient or family members of the patient's diagnosis and prognosis. If, however, family members requested that a patient not be told his diagnosis, the request was honored.

Understandings were more tacit, of shorter duration, and not usually as generalizable from situation to situation. They were unique to a particular patient unit or between specific interactors. They were broken or stretched as often as they were honored. For example, because one physician did not want his patients to "compare notes" regarding their treatments and progression of their illnesses, he insisted that they not be placed in rooms together. In addition, although not stated explicitly, it was generally recognized that he preferred that patients be provided only limited information regarding their conditions or their prospects for the future. These patients generally searched for more information; they usually pressed nurses and nursing staff for information about themselves and about other patients as they attempted to evaluate their own progress. The nurses did not place patients in rooms together but, believing that patients should have the information they were requesting, encouraged them to sit in the lounge where they would come in contact with other patients with the same illness. In this way they provided patients with access to the information they requested, stretching rather than breaking the understanding.

The appropriateness of alternative action or inaction was evaluated partly in terms of the outcome, not only in terms of the patients' and families' welfare but also in terms of its impact upon the health professionals. For example, the agreement that "only physicians tell families that a patient is dying" was simple enough to honor when viewed as an abstraction and when it involved only two groups, physicians and nurses. It was difficult to honor, however, in real interactions where there were other interactors—the patient, family members, friends—to consider and where there were other agreements and understandings to consider. One major agreement was that each health care provider is responsible for attending to the needs and problems of patients and family members. In a situation where the patient or family members pressed nurses for information and where the physician either did not want, or was not available, to provide this information, or where nurses did not know the physician's intent, the nurses were faced with the dilemma of which rule to honor. Nurses resolved this dilemma through a bargaining process which included weighing possible individual penalties and rewards if they should give the patient the requested information.

PENALTIES AND REWARDS

The penalties for acting contrary to agreements and understandings, either purposefully or inadvertently, were based on judgments related both to the situation and the outcome. Thus, penalties were negotiable. In most instances penalties took the form of chastisement or unpleasant confrontations between interactors. What constituted poor or good judgment depended upon ideology, hierarchical position, and professional background. A confrontation could follow honoring agreements as well as breaking them.

No interactors were immune from unpleasant confrontations. Generally confrontations arose from decisions which resulted in patient or family dissatisfaction or reflected adversely on health professionals. Such confrontations occurred in situations where interactors had not, for whatever reasons, arrived at a consensus about the situation and thus there was no basis for negotiating for mutually acceptable roles.

For example, Mrs. O., a 34-year-old woman who had had a mastectomy for cancer of the breast, was readmitted to the hospital for further treatment. She talked openly about her condition to physicians and nurses. The patient and her sister were watching a documentary about cancer in women on television. When the nurse entered the room, the patient made reference to the television program and then asked the nurse about her experience in caring for patients with cancer. In responding, the nurse referred to having cared for patients "like her" many times. The next day the sister confronted the patient's physician demanding to know why *he* did not control what *his* nurses said. It was her opinion that the nurse was "insensitive and cruel" to have mentioned her sister's cancer.

The physician, having no knowledge of what had occurred, was embarrassed by the situation and felt obligated to rectify it by promising the sister that such an incident would not recur. The situation might have been avoided if the nurse had been aware of the visitor's definition of the situation that mentioning the patient's cancer in the visitor's presence was taboo.

Actually, the physician's promise had the potential for creating even more conflict. It was an empty promise. The nurses do not belong to the physician. Nurses are accountable to the patients and to the nursing service of the hospital. More importantly, no one person, physician or lay person, can control what interactors will say to each other throughout the day. Moreover, the patient introduced the conversation, was comfortable with it, and would probably do so again.

SOCIALIZATION WITHIN THE HOSPITAL

Understandings and agreements were perpetuated by a continuous process of *socialization* which was both deliberate and incidental. Who became the socializing agent was more dependent upon length of time in a particular setting and prior experiences than formal roles. In essence, general competence related to a particular situation rather than legitimate authority was the determining factor. Prior similar experiences, ability to predict outcomes, ease of interactions, and knowledge of bureaucratic channels of communication were important factors in determining this competency.

Nurses played a primary role in socializing patients, visitors, and house officers, which was probably related to a number of factors. Nurses were permanently assigned to a unit and generally spent more actual time interacting with any one interactor throughout the patient's hospital stay. In addition, they were present more consistently during the process of dying and at the time of the patient's death. They were also more likely than other professionals to have been socialized in their educational programs to rules consonant with the care of dying patients and their families. There was, however, a great variation among all interactors. Nurses often socialized other nurses, as did patients and physicians.

The following episode was typical. It was 8:00 p.m. and most visitors had gone. The corridors were quiet and patients were in their rooms for the night. The nurse/researcher entered the room of Ted, a 20-year-old man admitted the day before. He was no stranger to her since he had been admitted to the hospital on numerous occasions over the past two years. He was the only child of elderly parents. His father was a stock broker. His mother, a college graduate, had spent the past two years caring for him at home. They were aware of his diagnosis and prognosis. Ted, who had Hodgkin's disease, had been told he had an "inflammation of the lymph nodes." His parents were vehement about keeping "the secret" and could not be convinced otherwise. Health care providers complied with this request but expressed their disagreement to each other.

Ted's mother saw the nurse/researcher walking toward Ted's room and hurriedly followed her into the room. She was fearful that someone would "tell the secret" so she accompanied hospital personnel whenever they entered the room. Most conversations with Ted in the past were directed through his mother. As a consequence, he was relegated to a passive role.

Conversation was not the issue at this point. Ted was moribund and would probably die within a few hours.

Mother:	Oh, it's you, I'm glad it's you. He's better; no he's not, but he's been sick before. You make him better, you can if you want to.
Nurse/Researcher:	I'll try to make him comfortable. He is very ill. I wish I could, but I can't make him better.
(Mother and nurse/researcher walk into the corridor.)	
Mother:	He's worse, is he dying? No, he's not dying . . . yes, he is . . . is he?
Nurse/Researcher:	Yes, I think he may be.
Mother:	Soon?
Nurse/Researcher:	Yes soon, very soon, but he is not in pain now, he is sleeping.

It was now 9:30 p.m. The parents were in the hallway adjacent to the room. The young man had died despite attempts on the part of the house officers to "help him." The nurse/researcher and the intern were still in the patient's room where they had been for the last 45 minutes.

Intern:	God, he's dead. I didn't expect it.

(The nurse/researcher looked surprised.)

Intern:	You knew it, didn't you?
Nurse/Researcher:	Yes, I'm sorry, I should have told you.
Intern:	Oh, that's okay. What happens now? You tell the family!
Nurse/Researcher:	Well, we'll make him look as pleasant as possible, get rid of all this stuff [hospital equipment] and then I'll come with you while *you* speak to the family. It's not unusual for them to cry out and run into the room and touch the body. It's okay if they do. I won't leave. She [referring to Ted's mother] will probably be quiet at first.
Intern:	Okay, should we do it now?
Nurse/Researcher:	Wait a minute until we get rid of all these needles and things. [The nurse/researcher intentionally stalled for time for her own as well as the intern's benefit.] I know this is a difficult thing for you. Take your time, they will probably know before you speak.

(The intern and nurse walked toward the family.)

Father:	Oh, no, no!
Intern:	(Mumbles) I'm terribly sorry.

Ted's mother remained seated in a trance-like state. Ted's father turned to his wife, stroking her and softly and gently said: "Mother, mother, what are we going to do? I don't know what I'll do without him. He was such a good boy."

The scene continued for what seemed like an eternity, but in actuality was only 12 minutes. The intern had gone; the nurse/researcher remained with the family.

Father:	May I see him?
Nurse/Researcher:	Yes, of course.

The nurse/researcher led the way to the room. Ted's mother, although walking unassisted toward the room shouted almost hysterically:

No, no, I can't go in! Ted, Ted, why did you leave me? Why did you go?

House officers and nurses hurried to the room. At this point Ted's father was in the room with Ted.

Father:	(softly and calmly) Come in Mother, Ted would want it.
Intern:	Get her out, hold her, hold her.
Nurse/Researcher:	(quietly to intern) Wait, see what she does, it's better for her to cry than that catatonic state she was in back there (referring to when she was seated in the chair).
Intern:	Yes, okay, will you stay with her?
Nurse/Researcher:	Yes, I will. Don't forget to call Dr. _____. He'll probably want to come back. (The private physician had left the hospital shortly before.)

This example demonstrates the deliberate socialization of the intern by the nurse/researcher and his acceptance of this process in learning how to deal with the family after a patient had died. There was first the explanation of what must be done, then preparation for expected reactions on the part of family members and approval of the anticipated behaviors. In addition, there was reinforcement of the agreement that it is traditionally a physician's responsibility to inform the family of the patient's death.

Rules of behavior arise in interactions and then become habitual. They become institutionalized to greater or lesser degrees as future generations are socialized to them. Multiple realities are socially created and then are perceived as objectively real. These realities are always in the process of construction in addition to being a pre-existing phenomenon. Roles are developed within these objective realities through a negotiating process.

NEGOTIATION FOR ROLES

THE CASE OF MR. W.

In order to discuss the process of negotiation, an example is provided as an introduction. The brief analysis following this interaction serves to orient the reader to the various influences which subtly affected each interactor, and to lend more meaning to the following discussion.

Mr. W. was a 60-year-old patient with cancer of the lung. He was single, a college graduate and former businessman. His only living relative was his aged mother who lived in another state. Two sisters who were friends of long standing had assisted him while he was at home, managed his affairs, and were his only "family." He had become progressively more ill during his hospitalization and at the time of the following interactions, it was clear he would die that evening. One of the women recognized the gravity of the situation and began looking for confirmation of her belief that he was dying. A house officer was responsible for the medical care of this patient in the private physician's absence.

One woman, the patient's closest friend, approached the house officer at 6:00 p.m.

Friend:	I have to call his mother. What should I tell her?
House Officer:	Tell her what is wrong with him.
Friend:	She knows what is wrong with him. I mean, what should I tell her?
House Officer:	She should know what is wrong with him.
Friend:	(exasperated) She knows what's wrong—I meant, what should I tell her!
House Officer:	Tell her the truth. (He turned from her.)

The friend walked away with tears in her eyes and returned to the room. She sat with the patient who remained quiet and in no acute distress.

The nurse/researcher and other members of the nursing staff overheard the conversation between the house officer and Mr. W.'s friend. They looked expectantly at the house officer.

House Officer:	(to nursing staff) Well, what do you want me to do? I don't know what's going on. I saw the guy for the first time today.
Nurse/Researcher:	I haven't cared for him before, either, but he looks really sick.
House Officer:	Yeah, but I don't know. She said he was this sick before and got better.
Nurse/Researcher:	Do you think that's a possibility this time?
House Officer:	(Shrugged his shoulders and walked away.)

The nurse/researcher turned to the other members of the nursing staff and asked:

> Have any of you cared for Mr. W. before? Does he look different? Is he acting differently?

Unfortunately, none of them was familiar with Mr. W.'s prior physical condition or behavior. He had been admitted to the hospital that morning. On his prior admissions to the hospital, he had been assigned to another patient care unit and was unknown to these nurses.

The nurse/researcher was in a quandary as to what and when to say something to this woman. The patient's prognosis appeared grave. He was certainly at high risk of dying, but was he dying? Should she tell the friend to call Mr. W.'s mother in Wisconsin? The nurse/researcher decided to talk with the two friends and to re-evaluate Mr. W.'s physiological status.

As she entered the patient's room, Mr. W. looked up and motioned to her. He did not speak but pointed to his mouth. It looked dry. The nurse/researcher offered him some water. He motioned her away and pointed to his mouth again. There was a glass of eggnog on his bedside stand. The nurse/researcher offered him some eggnog. He smiled and nodded yes. The nurse/researcher held the glass while he took a few sips.

He mumbled something. When the nurse/researcher asked him to repeat what he said, he said, "Dying is . . ." The last word was incoherent and he never spoke another word. He motioned for more eggnog.

The nurse/researcher tried to feed him his eggnog. He was obviously much worse than earlier in the afternoon. It was difficult for him to swallow. It was 6:15 p.m.

Friend:	Nurse, I would like to try.
Nurse/Researcher:	To feed him?
Friend:	Yes.
Nurse/Researcher:	Okay, you might try using this paper cup. Squeeze it like this, but don't be too disappointed if he won't drink; he is very sick and very weak and tired.

At 6:30 p.m. he looked worse; his respirations and pulse were more rapid and his blood pressure increased. The nurse/researcher instructed the friend not to try to feed him any longer and suggested that she come into the hall for a moment. She appeared distracted and on the verge of tears as she followed the nurse/researcher into the hall.

Nurse/Researcher:	I just wanted to talk to you for a moment.
Friend:	(nods affirmatively and looks fearful)
Nurse/Researcher:	(quietly) Do you know how very ill he is at this moment?
Friend:	I know what he has. He had radiation and he did so good for a year. I've seen him this sick before and it worked out okay.

The friend repeated the conversation she had with the house officer adding that she was not satisfied with the answer she had received.

Friend:	I don't know what to tell his mother, she is old and he is an only child.
Nurse/Researcher:	He is very ill at this moment.
Friend:	What should I tell his mother?
Nurse/Researcher:	Are you asking me if he will die?
Friend:	Yes, shall I tell his mother?
Nurse/Researcher:	He is very sick at this moment. He is not suffering and there is always the possibility that he may get a little better, but it doesn't seem likely.
Friend:	Will he leave the hospital?
Nurse/Researcher:	I do not think he will ever be able to go home again. It would be wise to call his mother.
Friend:	When will *IT* happen?
Nurse/Researcher:	That is very difficult to answer. If he continues to breathe like he is at this moment it will be soon.
Friend:	Soon! What is soon?

The nurse/researcher was sure the friend wanted the question answered, but she was not sure how soon she wanted it answered. The nurse/researcher remained quiet, thinking that if the woman continued the conversation she would tell her then; if the woman walked away she would wait a while. Either way, the nurse/researcher intended to tell her since she believed he would die before 8:00 p.m. The friend requested to use the telephone. The nurse/researcher placed the long distance call for her. The friend told Mr. W.'s mother that he would probably die. After the telephone call they returned to the room. The nurse/researcher told the friends she would return shortly but if they needed anything before she returned to ring the call bell and she would come. When she returned in one half-hour Mr. W. was unconscious. His pupils were unequal, left greater than right, pulse 142, respirations 44, blood pressure 200/100.

Nurse/Researcher:	(to friend) I think he may have had a stroke.
Friend:	You won't leave us alone?
Nurse/Researcher:	No, I'll just call the doctor and be right back.
Nurse/Researcher:	(to house officer who was on the unit) Mr. W. is poor. [She related the signs and symptoms and the possibility of a stroke; he shrugged his shoulders.]
House Officer:	So what—what do you want me to do?
Nurse/Researcher:	I know there's nothing you can do, but I thought you might want to look at him, more for the family's than for his benefit. Perhaps you could talk with the family.

House Officer: That's not his family, that's his girlfriend. [He was refer-
                   ring to the friend he had talked to earlier.]

Nurse/Researcher: She is all the family he has and she has cared for him
                   the last year.

House Officer: Okay, but there's nothing I can do!

Nurse/researcher and house officer entered the room. He told the friends to leave.

House Officer: (to nurse/researcher) You're right, there's nothing I can
                   do. Call me when . . . you know. . . .

Nurse/Researcher: (nods yes)

The patient became progressively worse. The friends became restless and acted like they did not know whether to stay or leave the room. His close friend reached out to touch him then drew back her hand and looked at the nurse/researcher.

Nurse/Researcher: You may stay as long as you like. I'll just put chairs by
                   the bed and you may sit near him if you like. You may
                   touch him, hold his hand, whatever you would like. No
                   one will stop you or send you away unless you want to
                   leave the room. Then you may sit in the lounge. I'll take
                   you there if you would like.

Friend: I want to stay, oh, I want to stay. I was afraid I would be
                   sent away. I am so glad you warned me. I am so glad
                   you warned me. How long will he be with me?

Nurse/Researcher: Probably less than an hour. He is not suffering; you see
                   how quiet and peaceful he is now. He is not working so
                   hard to breathe and he will just go to sleep.

Friend: He's not suffering? Oh, that's good. He does look peace-
                   ful. I'm so glad you warned me. I hoped it would be like
                   this, just sleep away, I mean. I was afraid I wouldn't
                   know, but you told me and now I know. Oh, thank you.
                   Now I know.

At 7:45 p.m. both friends were seated at the bedside. The nurse/researcher walked to the side of the bed from the foot of the bed where she had been standing.

She listened to Mr. W.'s heart, examined his pupils, checked for reflexes, then turned to both friends and said:

                   I think it is over.

Woman: I think so too.

(The nurse/researcher notified the house officer who came to the room to pronounce the man dead. The woman spoke first.)

                   I think he is gone.

House Officer: I'm sorry. I will call Dr. ＿＿＿＿.

The friend then asked the nurse/researcher some additional questions regarding disposition of the body, which were answered. The hospital mortician was called and came to answer more specific questions. After telephone calls were made, the friends turned to the nurse/researcher, and one said: "Thank you, thank you so much, you have been wonderful. You warned us and that is so important. Thank you for all you have done."

One friend reached out to shake hands, then the other friend took the nurse/researcher's hand and kissed it. They left and came back about five minutes later.

Nurse/Researcher: Did you forget something?

Woman: Would you tell us your name again, please?

The nurse/researcher gave her name. The friend repeated it twice, then nodded, stared at her for a moment, turned and disappeared onto the elevator. There was silence, although there were four nursing staff members standing and watching. The silence was broken by the house officer who said:

What time was it (he was making out the death notices)?

Nurse/Researcher: 7:45 p.m.

House Officer: Yeah, that's about right. I didn't check.

INTERPRETATION

Although this was a short interaction, lasting only 1 hour and 55 minutes, it illustrates the use of a hierarchy of rules. It also demonstrates the simultaneous, yet progressive, negotiating processes occurring between the various interactors related to their definitions of the situation, their identities, and their roles.

The friend first turned to the house officer, suggesting that lay people and professionals accept the revealing of this information as within the physician's domain. Notice the indirectness of her question in trying to define the situation. "What shall I tell her?" may be interpreted as "Is he going to die tonight?" The negotiating process between the physician and the friend was ended by the physician's response, "Tell her the truth" and by his turning away from her.

The opportunity for further negotiating was provided by the nurse. "Do you know how very ill he is at this moment?" However, the actual definition of his dying was allowed to emerge slowly. During this time negotiations for identities and roles were taking place between the physician and nurse/researcher. For example, the nurse/researcher approached the physician and confirmed her definition of the situation that the patient was dying and there was nothing the physician could do to cure him. Having established this, the rule was evoked that it was his responsibility to tell the family, "Perhaps you could talk to the family." His lack of conversation with the family and his request to be notified only when the patient had died further defined the roles in the situation. The nurse/researcher then had the option of telling the friends so that they could inform his mother. Through negotiating for roles, the nurse/researcher was able to achieve the desired outcome, the notification of the mother. The relationship between the nurse/researcher and the house officer remained strained.

It is important to note that even after mutually acceptable roles were established among all participants, there were additional rules operating. Neither patients nor family members were abruptly informed of the imminence of the patient's death.

There are many possible explanations, psychological as well as sociological, as to why the participants behaved as they did. Regardless of the explanations, of importance is that the negotiation for mutually acceptable roles and the choice of specific action or inaction is a complex matter affected by many extrinsic and intrinsic factors.

Generally, the process of negotiation began when health care providers encountered individual patients with specific problems. General rules for behavior were not directly applicable in individual situations or for solving specific problems. Consequently, all health care providers were necessarily adept at calling upon selected rules to achieve their own goals. They were also skilled at breaking or stretching rules when it was convenient or when a situation needed immediate attention. In either instance, choice of alternative actions or inaction was determined by the desire to care for patients or accomplish tasks properly as viewed from their own perspectives.

There was essentially a three-step process of negotiating with each step occurring simultaneously. The first step was to attain some consensus about whether the patient should be labeled *high risk of dying* or *dying patient.* The interactors then sought to incorporate into their performance in a particular situation those identities which were most important to them as individuals and which were not in great conflict with the expressive processes of other interactors. When these two stages were achieved, a working agreement was reached. Individuals then continued to negotiate for interactive roles based upon this working agreement. However, the working agreement or common definition of the situation was, at best, a delicate balance of interactive processes. It served as a set of boundary rules and as such governed the subject matter that could be included in a particular encounter.

Working agreements were far from stable as they provided only a beginning for negotiating for identities and roles. They were upset, revised, and changed as interactors struggled over mutually acceptable roles and identities that would be in accord with idealized concepts of selves.

FACTORS INFLUENCING NEGOTIATIONS

Many factors affected the interactional situation. Not all interactors negotiated from equal positions of strength. In general, health care providers negotiated from greater positions of strength than patients or family members. Age, diagnosis, and level of acuity of illness all influenced the opportunities available to patients for negotiating for roles. Interactors—patients, family, health care providers—who were unable to or were denied the opportunity to negotiate for roles, were relegated to specific roles by those interacting with them.

There were various sources of power available to all interactors. Possession of information, prior experience with dying, continuity of interactions, and interactions of long duration generally placed individuals in a stronger negotiating position regardless of their hierarchical position.

Before examining these factors, some cautions and definitions are necessary. The evaluation of positive or negative interactions is based on outcomes. Positive interactions resulted in the development of mutually acceptable roles based upon consensus. Consensus refers to the lack of impeding disagreements, and not necessarily to agreements on all levels among all the interactors. Although these relationships will be described in graphic terms they are, at best, observed trends since the nature of these data precludes accurate mathematical formulations.

AGE

There was a curvilinear relationship between the age of patients and their opportunities to negotiate for active roles. In other words, the young and the old had less opportunity to negotiate for active roles than the middle aged.

The role of young patients (under 20 years) was determined by their parents. Parents took great pains to deny their children access to information which would allow them to recognize or verify either the seriousness of their illness or their dying state. For instance, Paul, a 19-year-old college student dying of renal disease, knew only that he had a "kidney infection." Paul's parents, like Ted's, mentioned previously, insisted that he not be told the grave nature of his illness as they wished to protect him. Paul began asking questions and demanding more definitive answers regarding his health status. He expressed concern over whether he could return to school. Health care providers suggested to the parents that he be told the nature of his illness so that he could live as active a life as possible, including returning to school. His parents were vehemently opposed. One or the other of them remained in the hospital, following health care providers into the room, so "the secret" would not be divulged. When Paul asked direct questions about his sickness or his future, his parents told him not to worry "everything would work out." When he asked health care providers questions, his parents quickly responded by reminding him that they were there to answer his questions or by admonishing him not to keep the busy physicians and nurses from their work. Soon, Paul stopped asking questions. Even conversations not related to his illness were directed through his parents. The physicians and nurses grumbled among themselves about the injustice to Paul but did not intervene. As reasons for not continuing to negotiate with the parents on Paul's behalf, they stated: "After all, he's their son," "It's terrible and unfair for Paul, but it's his family's right." As a consequence, Paul was relegated to a purely passive role among the interactors.

Aged patients, usually 80 years or older, were also denied the opportunity by other interactors to negotiate for a mutually acceptable role. The aged, like the young, were relegated to passive roles but for different reasons. The interactors either interpreted the process of dying as an integral part of the process of aging or did not acknowledge the process of dying at all. These patients were described as "old and debilitated" and needing "attention and support." Their statements of "I am dying and I want to die at home" were frequently ignored or elicited responses, especially from family members and friends, such as "Don't be silly, you're all right," or "Stop talking like that. If you're not going to try, I won't visit you anymore."

SOCIAL CLASS

Although there were no observable differences in opportunities to negotiate as related to social class among the patients in this study, the comments and expectations of the house officers suggested there might be differences related to social class. It should be recalled that there were no medically indigent patients in this sample.

House officers, who had not taken care of private patients previously, frequently made comparisons between their experiences with these patients and those who were medically indigent. They raised objections to the private patients' requests for explanations, their criticisms of treatment, and their suggestions for modifications of their own care. It was not unusual for the house officers to describe private patients as "spoiled" or "non-compliant" and to suggest the need for more rigid rules and regulations regarding visiting hours and for greater control over granting patients' requests.

There may be other explanations for these comments and thus further study is necessary before any definitive statement can be made. The house officers' objections regarding private patients' behavior suggest, however, that patients from the lowest socioeconomic class may be accorded even less opportunity to negotiate for roles than those from other classes.

DIAGNOSIS AND ACUITY OF ILLNESS

Diagnostic labels influence the opportunities to negotiate for roles, both positively and negatively. For instance, knowledge of a diagnosis of malignant disease led to increased interactions and provided opportunity for negotiation if an early diagnosis was not interpreted as synonymous with dying or death. In other words, the interpretation of the diagnostic label contributed to the categorization of the patients as *high risk of dying, dying patient, chronically or acutely ill patient.* The high risk of dying patients had more opportunities to negotiate for acceptable roles than dying patients or patients in any other categories. The diagnostic label offered some structure to the definition of the situation, especially when there was a predictable course of illness or probabilities of recovery associated with a particular diagnosis.

The level of acuity of illness of the patient, regardless of diagnostic label, affected opportunities to negotiate for roles. Generally, the more dependent patients are on others for daily care, the less freedom they have to negotiate.

PRIOR EXPERIENCE WITH DYING PATIENTS

Another factor influencing the formation of mutually acceptable roles was prior experience with dying patients. Although prior experience influenced all interactors' opportunities to negotiate for acceptable roles, lack of previous experience was most apparent among family members and visitors, who continually searched for directives as to how to act or react to the dying patient. There are many reasons for this lack of prior experience. In addition to the fact that most people have not been present when someone died, dying was and still is a taboo subject. In conversation, the words death and dying are conspicuous by their absence. Lay people and professionals alike use substitute words or only allude to the fact that the patient is dying. Patients do not die, they "are gone," "pass on," "pass," "join God," or "expire." Patients are not dying, they are "terminal," "fatally ill," "won't make it," or are on their "last admission." Family members ask, "how long will *IT* be," or how long patients "will last," not "when will the patient die?" The taboo nature is reflected in the dependence on triadic patterns of communications, rather than on direct exchange of information.

Dying patients apologize for not getting well while family members express guilt feelings over their wishes that the patient die quickly. Family members describe these thoughts as "evil." They also receive conflicting responses from health care providers and lay people. Some interactors encourage the expression of these thoughts, interpreting them as normal and as expressions of love for not wanting the patient to suffer. Others describe such talk as morbid and discourage further discussions. The fact that these discussions occur at all and are encouraged by some interactors suggests a trend toward, or at least the desire for, more open discussion of dying and the development of skills needed to interact effectively with dying patients.

For instance, visitors and patients frequently ask nurses if they have ever seen anyone die. An affirmative response is usually followed by a statement or question as to how the nurse could "stand it." The following is a typical exchange which took place in a patient's room. The visitor, a woman, initiated the conversation as the nurse/researcher was about to leave the room. The visitor and her husband were seated at the patient's bedside. The patient had discussed her own dying with other visitors and health care providers on previous occasions. She was alert and listening.

Visitor:	Nurse, I would like to ask a question. Would you answer it?
Nurse/Researcher:	I will try.
Visitor:	Did you ever see anyone die?
Nurse/Researcher:	Yes, I have.
Visitor:	How could you stand it? I mean, it must be hard. . . . very sad. Do nurses feel sad when people die?
Nurse/Researcher:	Yes, they do.
Visitor:	Do they cry?
Nurse/Researcher:	Yes, sometimes they do.
Visitor:	Did you ever cry?
Nurse/Researcher:	Yes, I've cried.
Visitor:	About a patient?
Nurse/Researcher:	Yes, I have cried about a patient.

(At this point the visitor's husband became upset and motioned for her to be quiet.)

Visitor:	She's a nurse.
Husband:	So what?
Visitor:	She's a nurse, so I can ask her about dying.

She continued to ask questions about how nurses could stand to take care of people who were dying. She then said:

It's wonderful how you can take care of people who are dying. The worst thing about dying people is that it is so sad. Yes, it is so sad.

At this point the patient said:

It is not sad.

The visitors and the nurse/researcher looked toward the patient. There was a moment of silence and then she continued to speak:

Patient:	Sometimes people pray that they will die.
Visitor:	(Looking surprised) You aren't praying to die, are you?
Patient:	(Raised her eyebrows and shrugged her shoulders.)
Visitor:	Don't pray to die. We would miss you; we want you to come home.

Society does little to prepare its members for roles consonant with dying. In fact, socialization for the termination of any role is lacking. People are socialized to dying as a taboo subject. They know more about how to interact at viewings, wakes, funerals, and other events following death than about interactions with dying persons or their families.

The societal focus upon dying as a taboo subject leads to the avoidance of the topic of dying and to avoidance behaviors. This tradition of secrecy denies most people the opportunity to learn about dying. Because the subject is not addressed directly, learning is limited to those immediately involved. Consequently, individuals with prior experience are in a better position to negotiate than those without experience.

Interactors without previous experience enter the situation with preconceived notions which are usually negative, with fears regarding dying, and with vague ideas on how they or others should or would act. The inexperienced health professionals and lay people observed in the study recognized neither the signs of dying nor the possibilities for negotiating for roles. They were dependent upon the directions and predictions of more experienced interactors. Experienced interactors became the socializers and inexperienced interactors the learners, whether they were patients or health care providers. For instance, Cheryl, the 40-year-old woman dying of leukemia who had previously recovered from a catastrophic illness, socialized new nurses and physicians through her discussions of her prior illness. In addition, her prior illness served to introduce her to some of the expected behaviors accompanying the dying role. She was aware of her rights for special privileges and expected nurses to sit and talk with her. She rewarded this behavior by recognizing each nurse as an individual rather than as interchangeable cogs in a wheel. From her prior experience she became adept at negotiating for a role that was acceptable to her and those interacting with her. This acceptance allowed her to direct the behavior of others.

In the hospital setting, there is a continual process of socialization and resocialization even as people negotiate for roles. Health professionals, patients, and visitors were at the same time *agents* and *recipients* of socialization. Who became the agent depended upon the situation and upon the competencies of the individuals, not upon formal roles or hierarchical position. Thus, the socializing agent had greater opportunities to negotiate for acceptable roles than did the novice.

POWER

The fifth major factor impinging on interactional processes was power. The effect of power in the formation of mutually acceptable roles and role relationships was difficult to assess. Factors which were a source of power for an interactor at any one point in the negotiating process could serve to neutralize the power under other conditions, and might even change hands over time. For many reasons health care providers, physicians in particular, negotiated from positions of greater strength than other interactors, especially family members and, more importantly, patients.

First, the commonly accepted rules for interacting with dying patients gave the physician initial power over the nature and the content of interactions and

some control over whether interactions occurred at all. These rules were internalized by other professionals, in particular the nurses, who were responsible for
the day-to-day care of patients. The enforcement, or lack of enforcement, of these
rules by nurses influenced the opportunities available to patients and families to
negotiate for identities and roles acceptable to them. Secondly, since most of the
rules related to the control of information, information became a major source of
power.

Information. In the beginning, physicians had more information than other
interactors regarding the patient's diagnosis, available treatments and probabilities of success of various treatments. In addition, it should be recognized that the
first "working agreements" were established between physicians and their patients (and family members) prior to or shortly following admission to the hospital. In general, at least initially, the patients contracted with physicians for cures,
treatment, a return to some form of productive life, or freedom from discomfort.
Patients and family members expected the physician "to do something for them."
As one private physician explained: "Patients wouldn't come to me if they didn't
want to get better."

When the first contracts were made between physicians and patients, the
patients generally were not *dying*, although many were in the category of *high risk
of dying*. The expectations of the patient and his family were congruent with the
traditional role of physician, which is directed toward cure or maintenance of
health. All the behaviors or actions of the physician related to maintenance of
health or cure were acceptable to other interactors. There was little uncertainty
regarding each of the health care providers' roles and their relationship to each
other. As the patient's physical condition deteriorated, however, role relationships became vague. Patients and family members perceived an incongruity between their expectations for cure and a perceived lack of physical improvement.

Physicians were faced with a particular dilemma; their expertise lay in the
area of cure. Once it was established that there was no possibility for cure, there
was little in the way of guidance from pre-established norms and rules governing
their behavior or shaping the expectations of others regarding their role. At this
stage, physicians were expected to "do something" to prevent dying and, at the
same time, to promote dying with dignity.

Dilemmas arose when physicians either intentionally or inadvertently promised more than could be realistically delivered in terms of the patient's return to
a "more normal state of health," or when patients or family members misinter-
preted the physician's predictions regarding return to health, or when there was
no conscious attempt to revise the original contract with the patient or family
when dying became recognized as inevitable. When patients or family members
perceived an incongruity between their expectations for cure and a perceived
lack of physical improvement, they sought more information from the physician
regarding the expectations for patient recovery.

At first, interactions were not so much affected by the physician's revealing
or not revealing that death was inevitable as by the conditions impinging upon
and surrounding the event. The physician's revealing the information that the
patient's prognosis was poor generally provided the opportunity for open interactions with all interactors being free to negotiate for mutually acceptable roles. It
did not assure, however, that this would occur since not all interactors accepted

this definition at the same time or used the same criteria in defining that death was probable.

Physicians were guided by the medical model of diagnosis, available treatment, results of various tests, and their physical assessment of patients. Their actions were directed by their medical ideologies and their customary behavior with patients. For instance, surgeons relied upon available surgical techniques; internists (including specialists such as hematologists) relied upon drug therapies. Surgeons were apt to spend less time talking with patients and family members than internists.

Lay people and nonprofessional hospital personnel were more influenced by diagnostic labels than professionals. For most lay people, a diagnosis of cancer, leukemia, or Hodgkin's disease was interpreted as synonymous with dying. Generally lay persons had to rely on nurses and physicians for explanations of the meanings of observed changes in patients' conditions.

Nurses, although guided by the medical model, relied heavily on their own evaluations of the physical status of patients as observed in their day-to-day interactions. In addition, they relied upon physicians', patients', and family members' interpretations of a patient's status.

Withholding information confirming a patient's dying status did not assure that interactions would cease. If all the interactors were satisfied with the physician's communication, regardless of whether or not it contained the information that the patient was dying, there was a continuation of negotiations for mutually acceptable roles. This was at best a temporary state, whose duration was directly related to the maintenance of functional abilities of the patient and related to the patterns of living-dying. As nonimprovement or further progression of symptoms was recognized by interactors, there was a search for further information and confirmation that the patient was dying.

Confirmation of Dying Status. Figure 4 (p. 119) is a model depicting the effects of the physician's decision of revealing or not revealing the dying status of the patient to the patient or family members. It is also applicable to any interactors who searched for information and confirmation of their own labeling of the patient as dying.

Revealing that the patient is dying provides opportunities for open communication and freedom for all interactors to negotiate for a common definition of the situation, including the eventual legitimization of the label and mutually acceptable roles. Not revealing that the patient is dying, especially when the patient is actively seeking this information, leads to three possible reactions: (1) withdrawal or anger; (2) immediate search for more information; and (3) temporary satisfaction without search for more information.

Family, patients, nurses and other nursing personnel, house officers, and visitors respond similarly to lack of information but for different reasons. Nurses and other nursing personnel, and house officers (when they are not the patient's primary physician) express feelings of impotence, anger, and frustration over not being "*allowed* to tell." Family members express the same concerns over "not being *able* to tell" or "not *knowing what* to tell." In either instance, much of the anger is directed toward the primary physician, who is perceived by the other interactors as *unwilling* to tell, or *unwilling* to *share* information with the patient, nurses and nursing personnel, house officers, or family members.

118

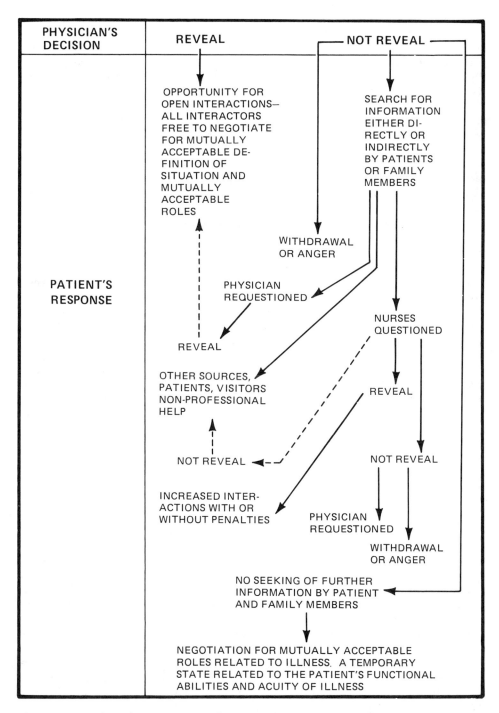

Figure 4.—Patients' Response to Physicians' Decision to Reveal or not to Reveal Their Dying Status to Them.

It is not possible to present the private physicians' view. Only six of the private physicians were willing to discuss the situation with the nurse/ researcher. All six physicians stated that their patients were aware that they were dying, otherwise their answers were evasive and noncommittal. Each stated that they would be interested in discussing the situation some time in the future when they were not so busy.

In their anger and frustration, most interactors believed that private physicians possessed information that was not made available to anyone else. Their view was fostered when physicians responded to their questions with silence or evasive responses rather than an "I don't know."

As can be seen in Figure 4, withdrawal or anger results in failure to negotiate further for common labels or mutually acceptable roles. When this occurs, individuals interact with each other in a ritualized fashion; their behavior is directed by expectations related to their formal roles, e.g., physician, nurse, and so on.

The second reaction, the immediate search for further information by patients or family members and other interactors, may result in direct questioning of the physician who then may or may not reveal the information, restarting the cycle. More frequently, patients and family members turn to nurses or other sources such as other nursing personnel or other hospital employees (tray carriers, housekeeping personnel), visitors, and other patients.

When nurses are questioned, they may or may not reveal the information. The consequences are similar to those described when the physician makes such a decision. Not revealing may lead the person to seek further information from physicians, other nurses or nursing personnel, or it may result in withdrawal or anger and decreased opportunities for negotiation. Revealing the information leads to increased opportunities to negotiate but may create a dilemma for the nurse who is forced to choose between two incongruent beliefs, "patients should have the information they request," and "only physicians initially tell the patient and family members that dying is inevitable." The nurse's disclosure of the information may lead to rewards or penalties, a process which will be described later in this chapter.

Of import is the fact that there is a reciprocal model that results from dissemination or non-dissemination of information that influences not only the behaviors of interactors but also their opportunities to negotiate for mutually acceptable roles.

The searching for and dissemination of information did not simply involve the physician making a pronouncement. Physicians, no less than other interactors, needed information regarding the health status of patients before they could make a decision as to their status. Although they had more information related to the probabilities of success of selected medical regimens, the probabilities gave clues, not direct answers, to predicting their success with any one patient. Uncertainty was a major factor in the diagnosis and treatment of these patients, especially when they were not clearly labeled as *high risk of dying* or *dying patient.*

As stated previously, no one individual in any interaction was able to define a situation and impose that definition upon others. At times, however, physicians had more power than other interactors because they assumed it or because it was granted to them by other persons.

Power, an Obstacle.   The power derived from the traditional role of the physician as the leader of the health team and curer of ills, was not entirely functional for the physician or for other interactors. For instance, when viewed as physician qua physician, the physician's opinions were perceived as edicts by patients and non-physician health professionals alike. Physicians, who recognized this interpretation, were reluctant to offer their opinions. The vagueness of their responses was interpreted as deliberate attempts to withhold information. As a result, the physicians received little support from other health care providers. This is only one example of how the bestowing of power alienates physicians as well as those who grant the power. Therefore, the formal role of physicians could impede as well as enhance their opportunities to negotiate for more acceptable roles.

This was no less true of nurses. Nurses were almost continually faced with the incongruity of believing that patients and families should have any or all the information they requested, and at the same time believing that, initially, only physicians could disclose this information. The situation was further complicated by the fact that disclosures of information held the reward of leading to open communication with patients and families and thus achieving the nurses' professed objectives as to what constituted the "best" care for dying patients and their families. At the same time, disclosure of information could lead to unpleasant interactions with physicians.

Generally, if nurses' disclosure of information regarding patients' status was favorable in terms of patients' or families' satisfaction, the incident went unmentioned, or was attributed to the unique characteristics of the nurse. If, however, a family member became upset by the information and complained to the physician, the nurse was described as "dumb," "incompetent," "stupid," or by the statement "what can you expect from nurses."

In addition, physicians, in particular those who evaluated their own successes and failures in terms of patient cures, were not averse to attributing progressive symptomatology to the "incompetence" of nurses. They had no compunctions about maintaining their own status and identity by degrading nurses and their abilities. More importantly, there appeared to be little recognition of the impact on the patients and families who were dependent on these nurses for care during the major part of their stay. The following example illustrates such a situation.

The patient was a 28-year-old male physician with a lymphosarcoma which rapidly led to his death. He had high and uncontrollable fevers about which his wife questioned the house officer. The house officer's response was to ignore the wife's question and to turn to a nurse and ask angrily, "How can you account for this? If you'd given the medications on time, this wouldn't happen. See that it doesn't happen again!" The nurse did not respond until she and the house officer were out of hearing range of the wife. She then said, "Don't you ever do that again. You know right well there's nothing we can do about that fever. He had his 'meds.' Why didn't you tell his wife the truth—what's the secret? If you can't handle the situation [the fact that the patient is dying], that's your problem."

Another example involved a middle-aged woman, also dying of cancer. In this case, the physician was the patient's private physician. The patient developed a very high fever and the nurse called the physician to see the patient. When he arrived, they walked into the room together. The patient was extremely ill but alert. The physician, in the patient's presence, turned to a nurse and said, "What are you trying to do anyway, kill my patient?" The nurse did not reply but the look on her face reflected surprise and disbelief.

She left the patient's room and described what had occurred to another nurse, saying, "What kind of a nut is he?" The other nurse replied, "He's always like that, don't pay any attention to him. He can't handle death, but he's a *good* doctor."

A third example more explicitly demonstrates the problem created by such physicians' outbursts. The following incident occurred in a two-bed room where both patients were extremely ill but mentally alert. Two nurses were in the process of weighing one patient. The patient had insisted on standing although the scale was constructed so she could be weighed lying down. Although it was more difficult for the nurses to allow the patient to stand, they decided to accede to the patient's request. As the nurses helped the patient to stand, her knees buckled and they had difficulty in supporting her weight. As they were maneuvering her back to bed, the secretary requested over the intercom that one of the nurses come to the desk to talk with a physician. Since two nurses were necessary to lift the woman back into bed, one nurse told the secretary she would be free to talk to the physician in about five minutes. About two minutes later an irate surgeon burst into the room. The nurses were still supporting the weight of the patient. The surgeon either ignored or was oblivious to the fact that the patient could have fallen and thus denied the nurse's request that he wait a minute.

Surgeon: I'm furious, what are you people doing, the chest tube on my patient is clamped. It has been clamped for 48 hours. I didn't know it was clamped. You fools don't do anything right. I'm furious. Who clamped it?

Nurse: I don't know, I didn't know it was clamped. How do you know it's been clamped for 48 hours?

Surgeon: You fools can't do anything right. You don't do anything for my patients. It's a wonder they survive.

The physician stormed out of the room. There was a silence, then the patient who had been sitting on the chair looked up and said to the nurses:

Did you really leave it clamped? Are you really hurting patients up here?

Nurse: He was just upset and wants the best care for his patients, and that's what we want too. We'll go down and see what happened.

As the nurses left the room, the same patient looked up and said:

Boy, he was mad, you girls had better watch out for him.

It turned out that a house officer had clamped the tube temporarily and appropriately after inserting some medication. When told this, the surgeon made a grunting sound, shrugged his shoulders and left the unit.

The above interactions may be interpreted in many ways. For purposes of this study, they will be interpreted as reflecting, in part, a negotiation for identity and control. Attacks on professional competence are interpreted as the epitome of insults by the recipients. The lack of a counter-attack on the part of the nurses partially reflects their concern for maintaining patients' faith in the professionals caring for them. In addition, nurses were aware of the dilemma faced by physicians who were ultimately held accountable for either continuing or discontinuing treatment for dying patients. The acquiescent behavior on the part of nurses, even in the face of inappropriate responses on the part of physicians (which were generally a display of authority or a means of enhancing their own identities at the cost of the nurses' identity) suggests the greater power base of the physician and perhaps the fear of nurses. Of importance is the fact that continual acquiescence led to the understanding that this behavior was acceptable. As such, it precluded further negotiations between physicians and nurses.*

The penalties to nurses were predominantly intrinsic, damage of personal and professional identity, disruption of established relationships with patients, and humiliation. The physicians had considerable potential power, at least from the frame of reference of the commonly accepted agreement regarding dissemination of information, especially when nurses interpreted the practice as a mandate rather than being open to negotiation. By interpreting the agreement as a mandate, nurses relinquished their right to make judgments based on the individual patient situation. Physicians then, to some extent, controlled the openness of the nurse-patient interactions and the patients' access to information. For instance, these nurses would respond to patients' and family members' questions by saying "You will have to ask the doctor." In view of the reluctance on the part of the family members and patients to directly question physicians, further negotiations for roles acceptable to them were impeded.

From the physicians' perspective, the unpleasant confrontations were not entirely inappropriate. In many instances, the success or failure of medical treatment depended upon the nurses' skill in implementing the medical plan. Generally, patients and family members attributed successes as well as failures in therapy to the physician. Failure of nurses to carry out the medical plan as ordered could lead to confrontations between the physician and family members.

Distressing encounters between physicians and nurses generally occurred when they reacted to each other in terms of formal roles and as strangers rather than on a person-to-person basis. When physicians and nurses made an effort to discuss the multiple factors in the situation, conflict was decreased. In situations where physicians and nurses had negotiated for mutually acceptable roles and where physicians had informed nurses of their unwritten contracts with patients and families, nurses were able to expand upon the physicians' negotiations in their interactions with patients and families.

Expanding Negotiations through Interactions. An interaction leading to expanded negotiations is depicted in the following. The patient was a 42-year-old woman dying of leukemia. Her pattern of dying was that of *peaks and valleys* (p.

---

*There is no intention to suggest that nurses are more concerned with patients' well-being than physicians, nor that this behavior is common to all physicians. The "outbursts" on the part of physicians stem from their concern for patients' welfare. Although there are callous nurses, just as there are callous physicians, nurses were not observed expressing anger directly to physicians in the presence of patients or family members. Although nurses express their anger to each other, it is unusual for them to confront physicians directly.

68). Both the patient and her family had known the seriousness of her illness from the beginning. The physician had also consistently shared his treatment plans and prognostic predictions with the nursing staff throughout her many hospitalizations. The patient was well liked by the care providers who were intrigued by this woman's ability to remain cheerful and concerned about other patients despite her own suffering. She frequently was observed walking up and down the corridors helping other patients with their meals or mail, or sitting talking with them. She would ask about other patients and their progress and respond by saying "Oh, I like that," or else, "Oh, I don't like that."

The following interaction took place on New Year's Eve just after a leave of absence to spend her "last Christmas" with her husband and children. She experienced some bleeding and telephoned her husband, requesting that he come to the hospital right away. Her physician approached the nurse/researcher in the hallway to ask about her condition. He said, "I just don't know what to do for her now. She is bleeding everywhere and not responding to treatment." The nurse/researcher then described her difficulty in evaluating the patient's condition. It had taken her 15 minutes to arouse the patient, and she thought for a while that the patient was unconscious when she suddenly opened her eyes and said, smiling:

Patient:	Oh, I'm so glad to see you. (She patted the nurse/researcher's cheek.) Did you have a nice Christmas?
Nurse/Researcher:	Yes. Did you have a nice Christmas?
Patient:	Oh yes, I went home for Christmas. It was the most wonderful Christmas of my life. My husband made it the most wonderful Christmas of my life.

A nursing aide entered the room and said, "Hello, Kitten." The aide then turned to the nurse/researcher and said:

	I always call her Kitten.
Patient:	I like that. (She then inquired about the aide's health and family.)

When the nurse/researcher left the room, the patient's husband was waiting for her in the hall. He inquired about his wife. The nurse/researcher told him she was not doing very well, but that she would telephone her physician so he could talk with him personally. The nurse/researcher stood off to one side while Mr. S. listened to what the physician was saying. There were tears in his eyes as he said "OK" and hung up the telephone. Mr. S. walked to the nurse/researcher and the following conversation occurred.

Mr. S.:	Dr. _____ told me that my wife was not responding to treatment.
Nurse/Researcher:	(Nodding) Yes.
Mr. S.:	What does that mean?
Nurse/Researcher:	It means that she is very ill at this point.
Mr. S.:	Does that mean there is no hope? I think there is hope!
Nurse/Researcher:	There is always hope, Mr. S. It means that the treatments aren't working at this time.

Mr. S.:	Why not?
Nurse/Researcher:	It is very hard to say. I know it is very hard, but we really do not know why she is not responding or if she will respond. She has an infection and the doctors have ordered the antibiotics I told you about, and now she has that bleeding which has slowed down but hasn't stopped. I wish I could give you an exact answer, but I really can't. I just don't know.
Mr. S.:	But what does not responding to treatment mean?
Nurse/Researcher:	It means that the treatment is just not doing her any good. It is not making her any better.
Mr. S.:	Could she die?
Nurse/Researcher:	Yes, Mr. S., she could.
Mr. S.:	Tonight?
Nurse/Researcher:	I don't think so, but I really don't know.

Arrangements were made for Mr. S. to sleep on a cot in her room. They watched the Guy Lombardo television show to welcome in the New Year. Mrs. S. looked up as the nurse/researcher entered the room and said "A Happy New Year to you. Isn't it wonderful, we had New Year's together!" Mr. S. did not answer. He followed the nurse out of the room and said "I know you [referring to the physicians and nurses] will stick with us. I just wanted to say I feel like the ball [on the T.V. program] was clicking off my life." Mrs. S. did not mention her dying until the next evening and then it was not in the presence of her husband.

This example illustrates the way in which the initial interaction of the physician and family members was extended, reinforcing and further clarifying the physician's definition of the situation.

From the example it can be seen that, although physicians could command considerable obedience from other interactors based upon their status in the hierarchy and their initial control of information, they could not achieve their goals without the cooperation of other interactors. In other words, they, too, had to negotiate, especially once relationships were established between the patients, their families and nurses, and nursing staff. Nurses, then, could have considerable influence since they frequently held an intermediary role between the patients and family members and the physician. In addition, they interacted with physicians and with patients more frequently and for longer periods of time than any other combination of interactors. This intermediary position of the nurse was recognized by nurses, physicians, patients, and families alike, as is demonstrated in the following situations.

The first situation not only reflects the recognition of the intermediary role of the nurse, but it also reflects the recognition of the possibilities of negotiating for desired ends, using a third person as an expeditor. The patient in this instance was also a physician. As a physician he was well-informed about his illness and had his own views on how he should be treated. Still, he recognized his role as patient and at times his behavior was threatening to nurses and at other times he expressed fears of his physicians. He related the following incident with pride. He was being fed at the time and asked for some salt which previously had been excluded from his diet.

Patient:	I can have salt now.
Nurse/Researcher:	Oh?
Patient:	Yes, I really faked them out.
Nurse/Researcher:	You did?
Patient:	Yes, I knew I was getting sodium depleted. I also knew that if I told the doctors, they wouldn't do what I said. So I had a discussion with the nurse and she was spokesman. I told her to suggest to the doctors that rather than giving me salt tablets, that they allow me to use table salt on my food. I even calculated the number of packets of salt that would be equivalent to a salt tablet. When the doctors made rounds and began talking about my sodium depletion the nurse said, "Well, how about if we replace that with salt in his food instead of salt tablets." They said, "Oh, that's a very good idea." [He then laughed and said] See, I got that nurse to do that for me. I knew they wouldn't do it if I asked them.

The second example illustrates the nurse's recognition of her role as intermediary between the physician and patient. It also demonstrates, in part, the effects of: (1) the patient's perception of the role of other, including the anticipated response and the impact of that response; and (2) the influence of nonverbal clues such as tone of voice and facial expression. Notice that the same question using the same wording when asked by the nurse/researcher and by the physician elicited different responses.

The patient appeared uncomfortable and distressed. She looked up but did not speak when people entered her room.

Nurse/Researcher:	How are you today? (quietly and without smiling)
Patient:	No better. I feel terrible. My leg hurts. I feel weak and I'm not getting any better. I want to go home before it is too late.
Nurse/Researcher:	Have you seen your doctor yet this morning?
Patient:	No, I am waiting to tell him. (Her physician entered the room.)
Doctor:	How are you today? (Smiling cheerfully.)
Patient:	OK, the medicine you gave me helps. (quietly and without much conviction)
Nurse/Researcher:	Why didn't you tell him you didn't feel any better and your leg still hurts?
Patient:	(Nearly in tears) I forgot. No, I didn't want to hurt his feelings. He thinks he is making me well.
Nurse/Researcher:	Would you like me to tell him for you. He *would* like to know.
Patient:	Oh, yes, you tell him. Tell him today.

ROLE CONFLICT: THE DILEMMA OF HEALTH CARE PRACTITIONERS IN FORCED CHOICE SITUATIONS

Physicians and nurses were frequently placed in situations where they were forced to make explicit choices between diametrically opposed norms or agreements and to act upon their choices. One such situation has already been discussed, namely, the nurses' need to choose between honoring the agreement that only physicians inform families and patients that dying is imminent, and their belief that patients and family members should be provided the information they request (p. 120).

There is another situation in which the norms underlying behavior are incongruous and thus create a dilemma for nurses in particular. This is the norm of professional detachment which is accompanied by the expectation that nurses respond in an unemotional fashion to unpleasant sights or events. The norm includes controlling facial expressions that might be frightening to patients or family members, or that reflect distaste or dislike of unpleasant tasks or an aversion to repulsive sights or odors. Nurses also advocate a humanistic approach in providing comfort or "TLC" (tender loving care). Although these norms are intrinsically incongruent, their disparity is amplified both by dying patients' wish for affection and communication through body language (note in previous examples the hand-holding and body contact that transpires between nurses and patients), and by the families' desire for "human" responses.

In the interaction between Cheryl's sister and the nurse/researcher (p. 87), the nurse/researcher initially thought that Cheryl had died. Cheryl's sister had accurately interpreted the change in the nurse/researcher's facial expression as an ominous sign. The nurse/researcher's ambivalence in evaluating her own behavior is reflected in her apologizing and at the same time justifying her behavior.

Sister: When I saw the look on your face I knew she was bad.

Nurse/Researcher: She's okay now.

Sister: You really care what happens to her, I could tell by the look on your face.

(The other family members were watching, there was a long silence.)

Nurse/Researcher: I'm sorry if I frightened you. We try not to change the expression on our faces when instances like that occur, but it is almost impossible.

Sister: This is the most wonderful place I have ever seen. The nurses are real people, and so human. You people really care about the patients up here. She had an attack like that this afternoon and the nurse had the same look on her face. It's wonderful that the nurses are so human and they care so much. I'm glad you had that expression on your face.

The following example demonstrates the negotiations for acceptable roles and identities when the interactors were forced to choose between two norms, equally acceptable but incongruous to each other. They are "the right of the patient to die with dignity" versus "the preservation of life and prevention of harm to patients."

A 71-year-old patient dying of cancer was placed on a respirator. The patient and her daughter, aware that the respirator was keeping the patient alive, later requested that the use of the machine be discontinued. The private physician told the daughter that he would come at 8:00 a.m. to stop the respirator. The physician then telephoned the nurses and told them to "discontinue the respirator." The nurses refused, stating that he should do it since he promised the family he would.

When the physician insisted that the nurses discontinue the respirator, the nurses contacted the nursing supervisor. She suggested that the house officers telephone the private physician to verify the order and that either they or the physician should discontinue the use of the respirator. An intern entered the patient's room to discontinue the respirator, cried, and then refused to do it. A resident physician finally discontinued the use of the respirator and the patient thanked him.

The nurses and intern in this instance agreed that the patient should be taken off the respirator; however, they *did not want to be the ones to do it*. The supervisor stated that since the nurses felt uncomfortable in performing this act, the responsibility remained with the physician. When asked if she would condone the nurses' following the physician's order if they felt comfortable about it, she said she would but not if the physician promised the family he would do it.

Under these circumstances it was generally accepted that private physicians were responsible for deciding if and when heroic or extraordinary means would be discontinued, regardless of the views of house officers and nurses. Private physicians usually made this decision in conjunction with family members and, less frequently, with patients.

In many instances the conditions of these agreements were not made known to other health care practitioners, in particular, house officers and nurses. In other instances house officers and nurses were aware of and honored such agreements. At other times they held private physicians responsible for acting on their own decisions, even in instances where they were in full agreement.

In this example, all interactors—patient, family member, and health care providers—were in agreement that the respirator should be discontinued and the patient be allowed to die. What was the problem? Why was each interactor turning to each other to perform the act?

There was no common agreement or understanding as to who performed this act. No one interpreted this action as part of their role. Nurses interpreted it as part of the physician's role. The private physician considered it a medical order to be carried out by nurses. Perhaps the tears of the intern reflected the incongruity of this act with his idealized concept of self.

After a process of negotiating, an understanding was reached and the resident discontinued the respirator. Only time and similar incidents will tell whether future health care providers facing a similar situation will use this incident as a model. If so, it may well become an agreement and a routine part of the resident's role.

SUMMARY

The situation of and surrounding the dying patient is characterized by:
(1) uncertainty and conflict created by the recognition of too many norms judged
to be of equal value; and (2) by the continual search for structure, bargaining for
rules of behavior, and negotiating for roles and identities.

Although there were rules regarding interactions with the dying patient
these were best described as agreements and understandings. These agreements
and understandings differed in terms of duration.

Agreements were long-standing understandings, which were generally honored and provided some structure to the situation, at least initially, especially in
regard to the division of labor. In contrast, understandings were less generalizable from situation to situation, and were broken as often as they were honored.
All rules were perpetuated by a continuous process of socialization.

These general rules for behavior were not directly applicable to individual
situations for solving specific problems. As a consequence, all health care providers were adept at calling upon selected rules to achieve their own goals or when a
situation needed immediate attention.

Essentially, the role developed from a dialectically related, three-step process
of negotiating. First, there was an attempt to define the situation in terms of the
label of the patient. Then, all interactors attempted to incorporate into their performance those identities which were uppermost in their hierarchy of roles, and
were not in great conflict with the expressive processes of other interactors.

The achievement of these two stages constituted a "working agreement"
which reflected consensus about the situation. The interactors continued to negotiate for interactive roles based upon the "working agreement."

The "working agreement" served as a set of boundary rules: (1) governing the
subject matter that could be introduced to a particular encounter; and (2) providing a beginning for negotiating for identities and mutually acceptable roles. It was
not stable. It was continually changed and revised as interactors continued to
struggle for mutually acceptable roles which were also in accord with idealized
concepts of themselves.

Not all interactors negotiated from equal positions of strength. In general,
health care providers negotiated from greater positions of strength than did patients and family members. Age, diagnosis, and acuity of illness influenced the
opportunities available to patients for negotiating for roles. In general, the influence of these factors was made more apparent as patients progressed along the
continuum from *high risk of dying* to that of *the dying patient.* Individuals who
were unable, or were denied the opportunity, to negotiate for roles were assigned
roles by those around them.

There were various sources of power available to all interactors. Possession
of information, prior experiences, and continuity and duration of interactions
generally placed individuals in stronger negotiating positions, regardless of hierarchical position.

In essence, there was a continual searching for structure, bargaining for rules
of behavior, and negotiating for identities and roles. Negotiations lead to further
negotiations. The common definitions arising from those negotiations were not
stable. They were continually revised as the situation and the patient's physical
status changed.

8   The Realities of Dying

In this chapter the presented findings will be elaborated on by raising new questions or asking old questions in new ways; by offering interpretations and speculative answers; by addressing theoretical and practical implications; and by identifying some practical problems and possible solutions to the problems. In addition, priorities for future research will be suggested.

WHAT DYING PATIENTS TELL US

Dying people live their dying in many ways. To understand a person's experience of living while dying, it is necessary to understand that person's perspectives on living in general.

The way people respond to the many stresses and crises throughout their lives influences their responses while living their dying. The competencies developed for living are the same competencies which are relied upon while dying. Just as people live their lives in unique ways, they also live their dying in unique ways. This is not surprising since dying is an integral part of living. To understand what it is like to be dying from the perspective of a dying person, it is necessary to know that person's perspectives about living.

DYING AS A PART OF LIVING

Although there are wide individual differences among people, there are also some commonalities. Generally people approach dying as they approach living. The knowledge that dying is likely or inevitable within the near future or within a short, predictable time period does not have magical properties. People do not suddenly or drastically change their behaviors or reactions, or their appearance, for that matter. Individuals who characteristically avoid confrontations in living usually avoid confrontations when dying. Chances are that stoic individuals will remain stoic, independent individuals independent, dependent individuals dependent, and so on. In fact, the knowledge that death is imminent may increase a person's need and desire to be more of whatever their previous style of living or behaving had been. For example, some individuals want to exert control and to make decisions regarding their lives for as long as they are able, while others prefer to have decisions made for them. Some persons may prefer to die in a hospital; others prefer to die at home.

Some individuals are very private—they characteristically keep their thoughts, feelings, and desires to themselves. Subjecting these persons to prying questions, thus stripping them of their right to remain private especially when death is imminent, is both insensitive and cruel. On the other hand, it is insensitive and cruel to deny more outwardly expressive persons the opportunity to share their thoughts openly and to make their desires known to those about them.

From the perspective of those living their dying, the cogent variable is the element of *choice, THEIR choice.* Are able individuals allowed by others and by themselves to live their dying in the way they wish?

THE ELEMENT OF CHOICE

The question of whether or not dying patients should be told of their fate was not of paramount importance in this study. All of them eventually learned of their fate. The circumstances under which they learned and the approach of the person imparting the information were of greater importance.

Patients described a system of filtering out what they did not wish to know or realize. They spoke of listening to or looking at the facts now, and then seeing or hearing them later. They expressed the need to have the facts permeate their thoughts at their own pace. They described reaching an emotional readiness when they suddenly heard or saw the facts and wondered, how long they had been there. Sometimes the facts needed to be introduced more than once by people around them. Sometimes patients looked for confirmation of what they saw or heard—of what they thought they knew.

There are patients who sincerely choose not to see or to hear, not to know. If that is their choice, then it is *NOT* appropriate to push them to know that which they do not wish to see or hear; that which they wish to deny. Forcing people to know, to see, or to hear that which they wish to deny is as inhumane as a conspiracy of silence about what they may wish to know.

The element of choice is introduced by fulfilling the need for a confidant who will initiate and allow dying people honest talk. The role of confidant is not an easy one. Talking of dying is not easy and periods of awkwardness and expressions of fear are inevitable. Patients were not looking for pity nor were they looking for consolation or sympathy. To the contrary, they spoke of their difficulty in facing the pity and helplessness they saw in the eyes of others. Patients looked for honesty and acceptance as they searched for understanding of their state by those around them.

They expressed their need for permission to die, the sense of the acceptance or at least the lack of denial of their state by those around them. This permission to die does not have to be spoken aloud. It can be demonstrated by visitors' and health care providers' ability to accept dying patients as people. It can be demonstrated through open and honest interactions and through continued care and caring. It can be inferred from tears or other expressions of grief or remorse when bidding farewell to a loved one.

The element of choice also lies in the dying person's decision to let go of their world as they knew it. That world includes every person and possession they hold dear. The ability to let go of everything one holds is closely related to the need for permission to die. Sometimes a caring loved one may honestly and sincerely need to invite the person to die.

The person whose family, friends, or health care providers deny him or her permission to die through their behavior or through their insistence on rigorous therapeutic interventions, despite ineffectual results, also deny the person the chance to let go of life. Those who are denied the opportunity to let go of life may die alone in cruel isolation since they are unable to share their burden with others.

THE ROLE OF THE DYING PERSON

Dying people describe their role in contemporary American society as being fraught with ambiguity, conflict and, in many instances, not compatible with the desires and needs of those who wish to live while they die.

Many factors contribute to this phenomenon. First, dying generally is not viewed as a part of living. Some people see dying as something foreign, as a state of oblivion or a period of suspension between life and death. Patients frequently negate a fear of death and they believe they are able to face death. Some even express their readiness to die. Yet, almost all patients speak of their fears of dying. They fear they will not die well, or that they will die in pain. They fear the unknowns of this new experience.

Just as some people live their dying, others seem suspended between life and death. Many fears and misconceptions are generated by the knowledge that death is imminent. The impact may be so extreme that their focus on dying precludes any emphasis upon living. As a result, some people cease all former activities and sit passively waiting for death.

In some instances other interactors relegate the dying person to a passive role. Under any circumstance a focus on dying rather than on living, coupled with the long-term nature of dying, compounds the difficulties faced by those who are dying. Stewart Alsop (1) described the time span between his diagnosis of leukemia and his death as a "Stay of Execution." Although it is an apt phrase, since it indicates the inevitability and constant threat of death, it also implies a preoccupation with dying. If a person is able to view dying as a chronic illness instead of a stay of execution, there can be more emphasis on living than on dying.

DYING AS A CHRONIC ILLNESS

Dying as a prolonged process assumes the characteristics of a chronic illness. Chronic illnesses have been described in many ways. The broad definition formulated by the Commission on Chronic Illnesses encompasses the major characteristics:

> All impairments or deviations from normal which have *one* or more of the following characteristics: are permanent; leave residual disability; are caused by nonreversible pathological alterations; require special training of the patient for rehabilitation; may be expected to require a long period of supervision, observation, or care (2).

Reexamination of the patterns of living-dying (Chapter 5) reveals the similarities in characteristics between living with chronic illness and with dying. All the patterns and possible combinations of patterns reflect the permanence of the emotional and physical changes of individuals as they experience multiple pathophysiological alterations. These alterations are permanent. No matter what the pattern, there is an overall decline. Each bodily insult results in residual disability and a need to accommodate the change. Regardless of the pattern, there is an observable loss of physical ability which requires prolonged rehabilitation, observation, and supportive care. The loss of physical ability can profoundly affect the person's behavioral responses and ability to cope.

What does this equating of dying with chronic illness mean to the individual who is dying? Dying people, like many persons who are chronically ill, express the feeling of being socially displaced. They talk about being alive but not being able to live. They grieve over the loss of former abilities and activities and they express sorrow over the loss of friends.

Some dying persons are no longer able to work, attend school, vacation, or participate in social activities because of their physical disabilities. More unfortunate perhaps, are those who are able to function independently but are deprived of these opportunities by the fears, prejudices, and misconceptions of people around them.

Half of the persons in this study had some type of cancer. Most of them recited anecdotes that reflected the societal stigma associated with cancers. Many of them were denied employment although competent and physically able to work. Some spoke of the broken promises of employers who were willing to give monetary compensation but were not willing to have them return to their jobs. Others expressed their sadness over the persons, including friends and relatives, who avoided them and their family members because of their fear that cancer might be contagious.

Like other chronically ill persons, the dying patients in this study felt somewhat suspended between the present and the future. They were hesitant to make plans for the future, even for the immediate future. When they did speak about plans for the future they were discouraged from doing so either by being told directly that their plans were not realistic, or indirectly by a lack of response from others or an abrupt change of conversation by others. Many of these dying persons expressed the sorrow of "desiring to do and not being able to do." Those people who survived beyond the predicted time period expressed regret over not having spent their time *more productively, doing the things they could have done then but could no longer do now.*

Changes in their customary life styles were associated with a sense of isolation which was intensified by frequent hospitalizations or the need to live close to medical care facilities. In addition, patients expressed a feeling of loss of mastery over their living situations. They expressed resentment, fear, and sorrow over the major changes in life style forced upon them by their progressive debilitation and by the attitudes of those around them about how persons should behave while dying.

DYING AS AN ACHIEVEMENT

The use of dying is another factor in shaping the role and actions of dying people. For many patients, especially those who had a prolonged course of living with dying, dying (especially dying well) became an achievement. These patients would speak of their dying and death on occasion to selected people but did not dwell on it. Some patients insisted on rigorous medical intervention, others refused any at all. Some of them insisted upon returning to their homes, their families, and their usual activities. Many of these persons were described by health care providers as being depressed or as denying or defying death. Perhaps they were, but careful listening to them revealed that they lived their dying the way they wished and thus from their own perspectives they died well. These patients did more than adjust and accommodate. They seemed to rise to an unseen challenge and in so doing expanded their living rather than extended their dying.

DYING AS A FAILURE OR SCAPEGOAT

A small minority of the patients perceived dying as a personal failure or attributed it to external forces. They berated themselves for their lack of past achievements. They not only faulted themselves, but attributed their state of affairs to bad luck or conditions over which they had no control.

A few patients also used their illness and dying status as a scapegoat. They spoke of all they would have achieved in life if they had not become ill. They frequently added "of course now it is too late to do anything [about it]."

Whether this small group of patients viewed dying as a failure or used it as a scapegoat, they exhibited a sense of futility and powerlessness. Some of them expressed overt anger toward their situation; while others appeared depressed, helpless, and resigned to their situation.

WHAT FAMILIES* AND HEALTH CARE PROVIDERS TELL US

The impact of the knowledge that death is imminent extends beyond the dying persons to their families, social groups, and society. In this study, family members and health care providers told of their perspectives about the realities of dying.

DYING AS A COHESIVE FORCE

Participation in the dying experience served as a cohesive force in some families and a disruptive force in others. In general, families who were unified in their everyday living situations or who had joined forces during previous crises offered each other strength and support. The stresses, strains, and uncertainties of the situation drew them closer to each other, creating social and emotional solidarity.

Some family members expressed remorse over the fact that a loved one had come face-to-face with death before they realized how much they cared for and needed one another. These families pointed to the greater social and emotional solidarity that they gained from their experience.

The stresses and strains of the dying experience served to sever further relationships in families where cohesion was tenuous prior to the dying experience. In these unsettled situations, patients more frequently were apt to use their dying as a weapon to control the activities of those around them than in cohesive family situations. Expressions of guilt were also more apparent.

DYING AS A WEAPON

When a patient used dying as a weapon to control the behaviors of family members, the result was resentment, anger and, in many instances, retaliation by not visiting the patient or only visiting for a few minutes. When dying patients used their dying as a weapon to control the behaviors and activities of health care providers, it had similar effects. Although the care providers continued to care for the patients, they expressed resentment and anger among themselves about the patients' behavior.

---

*Family includes the dying person as a family member.

The antagonism of family members and of health care providers was recognized by the patients who, in most instances, considered the behaviors of others as unreasonable for, after all, they were dying. The problem was lessened when the situation was addressed as openly and as honestly as possible but it was rarely resolved.

Whether the interactor was a dying person, family member, or health care provider, it was difficult to deal with the expression of resentment, anger, or long-term depression. When any chosen form of expression by any interactor was interpreted as an inappropriate response or effect, it was usually a signal of the interpreter's inability to cope. It was one more factor which contributed to the lack of understanding about the realities of dying. Another factor which impinged on understanding the realities of dying was the attempt to deal reasonably with what often was an unreasonable situation.

CAPTIVES IN AN UNREASONABLE LIFE SITUATION

Family members spoke of feeling like prisoners, captives in an unreasonable life situation. Each family member's (including the dying person) life-style was influenced to a greater or lesser degree by the physical and emotional state of the dying member.

The emotional tenor and activities of living surged and declined as the dying person's emotional and physical status changed either predictably or unpredictably. The degree of feeling captive increased as the uncertainty increased, and when the dying family member was at the lowest ebb of life. When dying persons were no longer able to participate in their own care by performing the usual tasks of daily living including feeding, bathing, dressing themselves, or turning over in bed independently, family members' feelings of captivity intensified. The dying person and the family member primarily responsible for the dying individual's care described feelings of being a captive more than any other interactors.

The actual physical demands for care are one reason for this feeling of captivity. Another reason is the difficulty of integrating or incorporating emotional or behavioral extremes into everyday living in a meaningful way.

All of the interactors—dying persons, family members, and health care providers—expressed similar fears and hopes. They described their grief over the many losses and changes in their lives. They recounted past incidents and events shared with the dying person. Reminiscing served not only as a reminder of what used to be, but also as a contrast for what is now and what is yet to come.

Not all evaluating of past events evoked pleasurable thoughts. Spouses spoke of their nagging doubts about whether their husbands or wives (whether the dying person or not) loved them still, or whether they ever loved them at all. The care-giving family members told of their loved ones' expectations for care and of their own increasing and, at times unbearable, emotional fatigue. They described their burden of sorrow coupled with their increased responsibilities for the dying loved one and other family members. They expressed fears of not being able to continue and of being abandoned by those around them, and hopes that neither would occur.

Family members who assumed major responsibility for caring for the dying person who chose to live his or her last hours and weeks at home at times

became overwhelmed with the enormity of the tasks they were expected to perform. Whether or not family members had prior experience or training or a desire
to learn to render physical care, administer medications, change dressings, irri-
gate wounds or ostomies, change beds, and all other tasks entailed, was not a
consideration. The general expectation of society is that the family will do so
because they should. It might be added that, with few exceptions, no other resources are available so they must assume the responsibilities whether they wish
to or not.

The lack of resources includes professional home care services as well as the
lack of assistance of friends. Family members were quick to tell of the numbers of
persons who offered to help but were always too busy with other things when
asked for assistance. They expressed resentment over the numbers of flowers and
plants received in place of helping hands, a listening ear, or a welcomed visit.

The pressures felt by family members, or health care providers caring for
dying persons arise not only from the expectation of others, but from their own
fears and hopes about the dying person.

PARALLEL FEARS AND HOPES

The fear of the dying person's being abandoned was a motivating force to all
in the situation. Family members took precautions to prevent their loved ones
from being abandoned, whether at home or in the hospital. They arranged for
someone to stay at the dying person's bedside. They pressed nurses and nursing
personnel for promises and assurances that the dying person would not be left
alone.

Family members frequently experimented with the call bell to summon
nurses and nursing personnel for minor requests. This action provided them the
opportunity to evaluate whether or not the call would be answered, the length of
response time, the availability, approachability, quality of care, and the caring and
understanding of the nurse or other nursing personnel. Nurses and nursing staff
were aware of the purposes of these actions. They sometimes became irritated by
them and expressed their irritations to each other. They understood the family's
behavior for they also feared that the patient would be abandoned by the family,
or health care providers. Physicians expressed similar fears. Physicians frequently
asked if family members had visited. They admitted to writing medical orders for
such things as unnecessary monitoring of vital signs to assure that nurses would
be with the patient. Family members asked if their physician had visited. Nurses
and nursing personnel sought reassurance from each other that someone would
care for *their patient* while they went to meals or when they were not present.
Each individual care giver—physician, nurse, nursing assistant, social worker,
and so on—saw herself or himself as the one and only advocate or protector of
the dying person. *Each believed that without his or her interventions the person
would be totally alone.* In reality many health care providers served interrelated
functions in caring for a patient. When the fear of each about patient abandonment was not recognized or was not shared openly, many misunderstandings
arose. Health care providers acted in anger toward each other and they dis-
trusted the actions and motives of others. They expressed feelings of lack of
support and abandonment by other health care providers. Each care giver felt
alone, overburdened and, at times, overwhelmed.

The fears of the family members and care givers paralleled other fears of the patient. They, no less than the patient, feared the diagnosis. Everyone in the situation waited with some fear and trepidation for the results of lab tests.

Persons, in general, feared pain. Each may have had a different perspective but there were fears of hurting, being hurt, or being unable to cope with pain, felt if not always expressed by all the interactors.

The literature is replete with studies of pain and pain management, as well as advice about the needs of patients, care givers, and family members. Yet, the problems and dilemmas associated with dying and death seem at times insurmountable. Even the language forces the use of terms such as the *dying person* or patient, *living their dying, living-while-knowingly-dying, high risk of dying*. There is no English word which encompasses dying as a part of living. But, the data from this and other studies suggest there is a need for more understanding of the realities involved in living while dying.

COPING AND THE REALITIES OF LIVING WHILE DYING

Attempts to understand and cope with the realities of living while dying are doomed to failure unless societal attitudes and the interactional setting are considered. The *interactional setting* includes the particular environment of care (home, hospital, school, hospice) as well as the individual characteristics, capabilities, and attitudes of all the interactors, be they the dying person, family members, care givers, or others.

To focus only on the needs, hopes, fears, and desires of people living their dying is not enough since the dying experience involves all persons in the interactional setting. The experience is a lonely and fearful one for all. Each person reacts to the imminence of death in his or her own way. Each has his or her own ideas of how and under what conditions a person should die and what constitutes a "good" death.

Multiple reactions and divergent views can and usually do lead to tension and conflict. These conflicts and tensions are usually acted upon but the causes are rarely if ever addressed directly. As a consequence, those involved may feel more and more lonely, more and more alienated. But, while dying is lonely, it is also a shared experience. In contrast to the many perspectives and divergent views about dying, there are common fears, concerns, uncertainties, and hopes.

Each individual in the situation copes with dying or deals with the situation in his or her own way. Yet, each is influenced by the actions and reactions of the other. Thus, the realities of living while dying cannot be understood or successfully addressed if focus is placed exclusively on the person who is dying without considering the total situation and setting. Although open and honest communication is helpful, there cannot be open communication if only the rights, expectations, and needs of the dying person are addressed. Attention must also be given to the needs, rights, and expectations of others in the interactional system. In addition, the needs, rights, expectations and responsibilities of all interactors must be addressed in relationship to each other.

Contemporary literature generally places the burden of initiating open, honest conversation about dying with those who have the most information, and this is usually health care providers. But open communication does not in and of itself serve as a panacea for the solution of problems or for making difficult decisions regarding dying people and their care. The literature suggests that if the patient is *aware*, there will be mutually acceptable solutions to problems and no need to hide from the situation. Although this may be helpful, it is only a part of the greater whole. Telling alone does not assure understanding or acceptance. Neither does it assure mutual reactions and interpretations. Each person in the situation has a prior history including a value system, attitudes toward dying and death, and established ways of coping with crisis situations. These values and attitudes are not the same for all Americans. Some are derived from different ethnic backgrounds and customs which are passed on from previous generations. Social class boundaries and ethnic barriers are difficult to cross, especially if differences are not expected in the first place.

Many other factors contributing to the ability to understand and to cope with the realities surrounding dying people and those who interact with them are not presented here because they are discussed in earlier chapters. For example, historical perspectives in Chapter 1; death as a social problem in Chapter 2; the sensitizing concepts in Chapter 3; characteristics of the interactors and variations in patterns of living-dying in Chapter 5; the impact of labels, labeling, and coming to consensus in Chapter 6; and the processes of negotiation, consensus, and socialization in Chapter 7. These factors will not be reiterated. In addition, there are other factors which may contribute to understanding the situation of and surrounding dying individuals and those who interact with them. These are discussed below.

THE REALITIES OF THE SOCIAL SETTING

This study was conducted in a medical center, an institution designed to cure illness, maintain life, and promote health. Common experiences with hospitals suggest there are rules and regulations to cover every act and occasion. Yet the data from the study revealed that there was continual negotiation for order and that hospital rules and policies were negotiable. There was a continual searching for structure, bargaining for rules of behavior, and negotiating for identities and roles as the health care providers were directing their efforts toward cure or maintenance of optimal patient function (Chapter 5). If this negotiation occurs in hospitals, it is likely that it occurs in other social institutions and life situations.

Several factors influence the negotiating process. Not all interactors negotiate from positions of equal strength. In general, physicians negotiate from positions of greater strength than other interactors primarily because they have more information regarding potential treatments, prognosis, diagnosis, and possible cures. In contrast, the patient negotiates from the position of least strength. Everyone who interacts with the patient, including family members and health care providers, can and does withhold information from the patient.

Information, not hierarchical position, is a key power factor. The power associated with formal hierarchical position is less significant than the power afforded by previous experience in interacting with dying patients. Prior experience gives interactors more knowledge about how to negotiate. Health care providers may have negotiated many times while it may be the first time for dying people or their family members. In addition, some interactors are provided more opportunity than others to negotiate for roles. The very old, the very young, and the very ill are least able to negotiate.

Socioeconomic status, religion, or ethnicity did not affect either the strength of the interactor's negotiating position or the opportunities to negotiate. Since there were no medically indigent patients in this study, information regarding the effects of socioeconomic status on negotiation is incomplete. Data on educational background was incomplete, thus it was not possible to evaluate its effects on negotiating behavior.

As the patient begins to be labeled the *dying patient*, interactions and opportunities to negotiate increase, but once the dying label is applied, the interactions change. Patients are accorded more privileges which they are expected to accept since they are dying. They no longer have the opportunity to negotiate for roles associated with living. They are expected to be passive, to not "fight to live," to not speak in futuristic terms, and to die within the expected time. Interactors are expected to adjust their schedules and life styles to meet what they perceive as the comfort needs of the dying patient for a limited period of time.

When patients do not die on schedule and do not recover, their opportunities to negotiate are reduced to almost zero. Interactors are released from the expectations associated with interacting with the dying patient and confusion arises as to how to terminate role relationship. Usual visits by friends or family members may cease and eventually the patient may die alone or with only a member of the nursing staff in attendance. This withdrawal may be attributed to the lack of socialization for terminating any role. Similarly, there is no identifiable, deliberate, anticipatory socialization to the dying role. Although most persons in the study had preconceived notions about dying, their specific roles and role expectations evolved through negotiation as they attempted to define the situation and their relationships with each other.

Conflicts between interactors were inevitable. They arose as a result of the process of negotiating and from the existence of multiple and conflicting norms. The existence of and adherence to potentially conflicting norms, none of which took precedence over the other in directing behavior, created role strain* for physicians, nurses, patients, and visitors.

Health care providers were continually confronted with choosing between acting on the norm of preserving life and preventing harm to patients, and that of allowing patients to die with dignity. This choice created role strain for all, especially in situations where patients or family members request that a patient be allowed to die, but the physician chooses to continue medical treatment. Under these circumstances nurses must choose between the conflicting norms of carrying out the physician's medical orders or acting as an advocate on behalf of the family. Acting contrary to the physician's wishes violates traditional physician-nurse relationships and may invoke the wrath of the physician. Not acting as an

---

*As defined by William J. Goode, role strain is a feeling of difficulty or stress in fulfilling the demands of one's role obligations. George A. Theodorson and Achilles G. Theodorson, *A Modern Dictionary of Sociology*, New York: Thomas Y. Crowell Company, 1969.

advocate for the patient or family is associated with a sense of guilt and failure and may discredit a nurse in the eyes of patients, their families, and other nurses.

Role strain also arises from the incongruity created by the traditional emphasis upon professional detachment and the goal of personalized care. Dying patients and their families are comforted by and reward nurses for a warm, individualized, and informal approach, which includes the use of first names, nurses' revealing personal interests, sharing their lives, and an overt display of feeling. In contrast, the traditional norms call for cool detachment and formalized interactions. Nurses, and other professional health care providers, including physicians, may be criticized for being "too cool and too detached" as well as for being "too emotionally involved."

Dying people and their family members are not exempt from role strain. The plight expressed by people trying to live their dying and by their family members are examples of role strain.

Conflicting norms and desires contribute to role strain for all interactors. Some of these conflicts can be resolved through a process of negotiation between and among interactors. For people to negotiate, especially patients and family members, they must realize that the situation is negotiable.

Competence in negotiating for mutually acceptable roles is gained throughout living. Skill in negotiating is not something which can be expected to arise when an individual is confronted with imminent death. It is a way of living. Negotiating abilities are learned, as are other skills, throughout the life cycle. One way to assist people in living and thus in living their dying, is to assist them in developing competence in negotiating throughout their lives.

Since many persons have not gained skills in negotiating, dying people, especially those in hospitals, may have to be told directly how to negotiate and what about their role and situation is negotiable. They may need to be assisted in manipulating the situation and the health care providers to meet their own needs.

Health care providers can assist dying people by maximizing their capacities to negotiate situations for a role more compatible with their life-styles. People's capacities can be maximized by restoring their power to control. Control over one's style of responding may or may not entail actively participating in and directing one's care. It may mean regressing or depending upon others.

The question remains, how can this restoration of power and continuity between dying and living experiences be accomplished? The question can be answered on many levels. At the broadest level, the answer lies in conceptualizing dying as a part of living. Secondly, the answer lies in recognizing the complexities of each situation and accepting that there is *no one best* solution to the problems encountered.

The primary task is to respond to *each* individual's actual dying experience. This response entails identifying the crisis and related stress at a specific time and responding to it and the emotions generated by it. It entails responding to where people are in their living as well as where they are in their dying. It entails more than summary information about the patient's world taken from a medical record, nursing notes, or word of mouth. *The task entails responding to each individual's dying experience as he or she lives it. Such a response precludes forcing any person to conform to preconceived notions of what dying entails or how any person should live their dying.*

SOME THEORETICAL FINDINGS

LABELING

Studying dying exposed labeling as an indeterminate, dialectical, perpetually unfinished process. The label of dying is not derived after one incident and it is far from permanent. The label itself arises through interaction. As Erickson (3) noted, there are three levels of analysis in terms of the audience: society at large; persons with whom the labeled individual interacts daily; and official and organizational agents of control. This study suggests the importance of a fourth audience, the individual who labels himself or herself. Although the three audiences may label an individual and attempt to impose rules of behavior based upon this label, it is not until he or she is aware of the labels and labels himself or herself that interactions are affected. This is not a phenomenon unique to dying patients; it is no less true, for example, of students who are labeled as "dull" or "bright." Based upon the findings of this study, it appears that the most significant changes in interaction occur, not when the patient is initially diagnosed but when the patient confirms the label in discussion with others.

ROLES AND IDENTITIES

Although this study focused on the dying patient in answering the questions regarding formation of roles at the interactional level, the findings are not limited to those who are dying. The findings are generalizable to other situations where there is questioning of social norms since individual standards for behavior are not separate from societal standards.

In the following discussion, social norms are viewed as part and parcel of Berger and Luckman's *objective reality* (4) (Chapter 3). As such, they furnish the social framework or superstructure of society. For instance, norms shape behaviors ranging from the way people talk, dress, and worship to the way they think and deal with dying and death. Although these norms are patterned in many ways, they are localized as to time and place. For example, norms vary across social classes, in different generations, and even in different sections of the same institution, such as the hospital. The norms are socially constructed and then perceived as real. Just as the norms are socially constructed so are the social values which accompany them. Social values tell individuals what they should think about norms. They are abstract principles of behavior to which individuals feel a strong, emotionally toned commitment and as such provide a standard for judging acts and goals. They are often regarded as absolute, but they arise and are disseminated through social interactions.

When norms are stable and unquestioned, individuals can securely "place" themselves in society and begin to take their role and status for granted. When norms are in question, individuals become more conscious of their own roles and the discrepancies of overlapping of roles become more apparent. For example, when an individual finds that his or her reality does not coincide with that perceived by others in the situation, it causes confusion and anxiety. In addition, the individual's behavior may be seen as defiant and as such may incur possible sanctions by others. Although this may occur at any time, in situations associated with taboos, such as dying, or in other situations to which people have been denied access, individuals are forced to negotiate for mutual realities since typifications are misleading or absent. Conflict during these encounters is inevitable:

In sum, in indeterminate situations, as exemplified by that of the dying patient where the norms do not fit, the indeterminacy exacerbates the lack of fit. It is conceivable that this finding applies in situations involving members of minority groups such as blacks, women, students, or consumers, and all members of social movements. The current focus of attention on the subject of dying may be viewed as a norm-oriented social movement as described by Smelser (5).

BEHAVIORS TOWARD DYING AS A NORM-ORIENTED MOVEMENT

"A norm-oriented movement is an attempt to restore, modify, or create norms in the name of a generalized belief (6)." It involves "elements of panic (flight from existing norms or impending normative changes), craze (plunge to establish new means), and hostility (eradication of someone or something responsible for evils (7))."

At present there is a concerted effort on the part of segments of society, such as journalists, selected members of various health professions (psychologists, nurses, physicians, and social workers), and producers of mass media (television, newspapers), to alter the taboo nature of the subject of dying and death, if not society's beliefs toward death and their actions towards the dying. This effort can be viewed as a norm-oriented movement in its incipient stages since persons involved have some degree of commitment to the change espoused.

This effort, which arose relatively spontaneously, is associated with a great deal of emotional fervor. It was heralded for the health professionals by the work of Kubler-Ross. The effort is associated with informal sanctions for behavior regardless of whether an individual conforms to the traditional pattern of not talking about dying or to the currently popular standard of dealing openly with the subject.

Because of the conflicting standards between traditional and new, any interactor may be a hero one moment and a villain the next, depending upon the social reality of other interactors, as is true in any social movement. For example, in this study, one physician invested considerable time and effort in assisting a patient to prepare for her death by granting her last requests, including her wish to die at home. He was applauded by advocates of the new standard for his sensitivity and criticized for his poor judgment by those conforming to the traditional view.

In the situation of and surrounding the dying individual, there is not only negotiating about relationships whether or not there are formalized role expectations; but there is, in addition, a concerted effort to reconstruct social reality. In the new social reality, dying is not the "catastrophe of catastrophes" and it is not only good but right to discuss dying and death and to do so with dying patients. In the hospital this effort is mediated by organizational factors, such as the autonomy of professionals, and at the interactional level by face-to-face communications that provide an opportunity to negotiate for a common definition of the situation.

COMMON DEFINITIONS: COMPARISONS WITH
McCALL AND SIMMONS, AND GOFFMAN

Presently there is some controversy in the literature regarding the significance of the common definition of the situation upon the entire interactional
structure. McCall and Simmons (8) (Chapter 3) propose two sequential stages in
bargaining; the negotiation of social identity and the negotiation of interactive
roles. They suggest that a common definition of the situation or "working agreement" is reached when the cognitive processes of the interactors with respect to
social identities are not in great conflict. The working agreement serves as the
beginning for negotiating the interactive roles. It is subject to change as the factors
in the situation change. Further, a single encounter may present the appearance
of successive phases of interaction, each marked by the negotiation of a new
working agreement.

Goffman (9) (Chapter 3), in contrast, suggests that boundaries are set by
transformation rules which govern the subject matter that can be admitted to a
particular encounter. The *transformation rules* and the *identities* of the participants make up the common definition of the situation. The tension from non-
adherence to the rules must be dealt with since a threat to the rules is a threat to
the entire structure of the encounter.

The findings from this study are not congruent with either McCall and Simmons' or Goffman's formulations. The definition of the situation *initially* served as
a set of boundary rules. The rules were stretched and broken; however, as often
as not they were followed without threatening the entire structure. In addition,
the common definition of the situation was continually revised as interactors
changed or as interactors revised their hierarchy of role identities and as the label
of the patient changed.

Unlike McCall and Simmons, three, not two, components were identified in
the bargaining process. Each interactor attempted to: (1) label the patient;
(2) place one another in social categories, e.g., nurse, physician; and (3) incorporate into his or her performance those identities which were uppermost in his or
her hierarchy of roles and yet not in great conflict with the expressive processes
of other interactors. These components constituted the common definition
which served (1) as an *initial* set of boundary rules which governed the subject
matter that could be admitted to the particular encounter, and (2) as guidelines
for negotiating for mutually acceptable roles. This common definition was not
stable; it was continually revised and upset as the components fluctuated (Chapter 7).

One could argue that labeling the patient as dying is analogous to socially
categorizing the person and thus, there are two phases as McCall and Simmons
suggest. If so, the categories would be dying person and living person; however,
dying persons as well as living persons are physicians, lawyers, and laborers.
Consequently, these categories are not particularly useful in directing behavior.
One also can argue that being labeled the *dying patient* creates a social identity.
This is an area of study in itself; but if dying leads to a social identity, one would
need to explore the effects of unstable or poorly defined identities on the bargaining process.

More important than the number of components of the process is the finding that the processes of bargaining are not sequential as postulated by McCall and Simmons. Rather, the processes are dialectically related in the sense that the processes of labeling or categorizing, arriving at a common definition of the situation, and forming interactive roles are contrasting but simultaneous; each occurs continually and each affects and changes the other.

The similarities and differences of these three interpretations suggest the need for further study of the process of negotiating. For instance, what are the effects of discrepancies regarding identities upon the process of negotiating for mutually acceptable interactive roles? It may be that where there is a priori consensus about how a person is categorized socially (physician, truck driver, welfare recipient, vagrant) and in terms of related identities and expected behaviors, the breaking of rules is more disruptive and threatening to the structure than where consensus does not exist. As a consequence, there may be less opportunity to negotiate for mutually acceptable roles than under conditions where there is little a priori consensus.

On the other hand, one could hypothesize that there is a curvilinear relationship between the degree of structure (where structure refers to a priori consensus or who the person is in terms of social categories and related identities) and opportunities to negotiate for mutually acceptable roles. High consensus and low consensus result in less opportunity to negotiate.

Although this study was conceptualized in terms of labeling, role formation, and the development of a common definition of the situation, the findings suggest that studying dying persons using Goffman's concept of stigmatization might offer further explanation. The term stigma refers to an attribute that is deeply discrediting. Possession of an attribute that stigmatizes one possessor can confirm the usualness of another. The attribute is neither creditable nor discreditable as a thing in itself. For example, educational achievement may be perceived as crediting or discrediting in different occupational settings. In situations where a college degree is an expectation, some workers without degrees may be reluctant to reveal this lack for fear of being considered outsiders or less competent than those with degrees. Others may flaunt the fact that they have succeeded despite not having a degree.

In contrast, in situations where it is not usual to have college degrees, degree holders may be reluctant to reveal their academic accomplishments for fear of being considered an outsider or a failure for not using their degrees appropriately.

When considering the two labels *high risk of dying* and the *dying patient* as described in this study (Chap. 6), there are two points to be made. First, these labels evolved within the context of the environment of the hospital where illness is commonplace and dying is expected. The interactional process and the inferences drawn from behaviors which led to these labels may differ outside this environment. Second, high risk of dying may be, in part, a biomedical label in the hospital; however, it may be entirely a social label when the individual interacts with "normals" in the world outside of the hospital. For instance, patients in this study who were labeled as *high risk of dying* by virtue of their diagnoses, were refused employment or forced into early retirement although they were physically able to work. Goffman describes society's attitude toward stigmatized individuals as one of benevolence; these individuals are treated as though they are not quite human and their unanticipated behaviors are attributed to the stigma-tizing trait. His concept of stigma applies to the dying persons in the study in that any unusual or unanticipated behavior was attributed to their dying state. These dying persons were looked upon with benevolence, but it did not extend to their life-style. Other interactors placed restrictions on their activities and thus on their ways of living.

Dying may be a stigma, just as blindness, physical deformity, or mental aber-rations. Thus, looking at the problem in terms of Goffman's concept of stigmatization may be a useful alternative for explaining the differences in behav-ior among dying patients and those interacting with them.

TRIADIC PATTERNS, CONFIDANTS, AND STRANGERS: COMPARISONS WITH SIMMEL

As described in Chapter 6, communication occurred in a triadic or a series of triadic patterns. Health care providers, patients, and family members did not always communicate directly with one another. Generally, one person served as an intermediary and as a facilitator or blocking agent in the transmission of infor-mation.

One can hypothesize from the data that when an interactor evolves as an intermediary and confidant, there is increased opportunity for interactors to ne-gotiate for labels, roles, and common definitions and increased stability in the interactional system. Conversely, when no interactor becomes a confidant or in-termediary, opportunities for interactors to negotiate for labels, roles, and com-mon definitions are decreased, or even negated, with a consequential instability of the interactional system.

Some comments on the role of confidant are necessary. It was stated earlier (p. 90) that this role is assumed by or bestowed upon a health care provider. The selecting person perceives the confidant as not needing protection and expects the confidant to act as an emotional buffer between family members and the patient. The selected person is cast in a role similar to that of Simmel's (10) stranger, in the sense that confidants are people who "come today and will stay tomorrow." They are not perceived as needing protection for they are at "the same time near and yet far." The confidant, as the stranger, is at the same time *in* the group but not truly *of* the group. This nearness and remoteness gives the stranger, in this case the confidant, the character of objectivity.

Family members and dying patients feel free to disclose information to the confidant that they would not normally disclose to other persons. However, the stranger-confidant is expected to transmit information between and among other interactors. The role of a mediary in triadic relationships is not new (11). What is new is the notion of a combined role of mediary and stranger embodied by one individual, the confidant. Data from this study suggest that there is inherent personal conflict in such a role, which simultaneously demands concern and objectivity. It also suggests the need for interactors to be socialized to this role.

AWARENESS: COMPARISONS WITH GLASER AND STRAUSS

As Glaser and Strauss (12) demonstrated, the interactions which transpire between dying patients and others is guided by their *awareness* of the *dying state* (Chapter 3). Because awareness is a cogent variable, the effect of social factors upon levels of awareness warrants exploration. As discussed previously (p. 117), information was identified in this study as a key power factor in negotiating for roles. It was anticipated that social factors such as ethnicity and social class would influence the level of awareness of the *dying state* by the patient and other interactors and, in turn, would influence opportunities to negotiate for roles.

Data from this study did not reveal observable differences in social factors such as religion, ethnicity, or social class and levels of awareness. It should be re-emphasized that since there were no medically indigent patients in the sample, the information regarding the effects of social class is, at best, incomplete. Replication of the study using a population of medically indigent patients is needed to determine whether or not social class has an influence on levels of awareness.

Although data about educational background were incomplete, they suggest that patients with higher educational levels did not press for more information leading to earlier awareness than did their counterparts with less education; this finding, however, is not definitive. Further study is necessary to evaluate the effects of educational status and the seeking of additional information which would lead to awareness.

Glaser and Strauss (13) also categorized the "transitional statuses" that define a person's passage from living to dying, based on the distinctions medical personnel make in viewing death expectations. Although the phrase transitional statuses suggests a continuum, their categories are actually a typology. Data in the study revealed that medical personnel do recognize Glaser and Strauss' four distinctions: (1) instances where there is question as to whether the individual will live or die and medical personnel are unable to predict when the question will be resolved; (2) uncertainty about death but there is no known time when the question will be answered; (3) death is inevitable but the exact time it will occur cannot be predicted; and (4) death is certain and the time of death can be predicted. Although these ideal types are serviceable in sensitizing social scientists, they are too refined to be of practical use to health care providers. Health care providers used two working labels, *high risk of dying* and the *dying patient* in day-to-day interactions. They label persons in Glaser and Strauss' first three categories as *high risk of dying*. When interactors agree that death is inevitable and the time of death can be predicted, they label the person as the *dying patient*. These two labels, which evolved through interactional processes, then became functional in influencing the interactional processes through which they arose.

SOME PRACTICAL IMPLICATIONS

The patients in this study initially negotiated for information and then consistently focused upon cures and treatment possibilities, even while they confirmed that they recognized they were dying. Many of the patients and their family members reached a stage of resignation; none was observed to reach the stage of acceptance which Kubler-Ross describes as a peaceful state, void of feeling (14).

COMPARISONS WITH KUBLER-ROSS

The practical implications of this contrast come in the application and potential consequences of Kubler-Ross's work. *Premature* labeling of a patient as the dying patient, either by misinterpretation of diagnosis or conversations of interactors which focused upon *dying* to the *exclusion* of possibilities of *living*, led toward *negotiating* for a *reality* that did *not exist.*

This is not to deny the importance of open discussion of dying or the provision of opportunities for patients to gain desired information. It does suggest that these discussions require an appropriate relationship between interactors be established first, and that the discussion be based upon the *reality* of the situation.

The superimposition by interactors of any model, such as Kubler-Ross's stages of dying, without an exchange between interactors which leads to a common definition of the situation as it exists in reality, imposes an artificial structure on the situation of the dying person. Thus, behaviors become ritualistic and may or may not be appropriate to what is taking place or is in the best interests of the dying person or family members. Further, *ritualistic* behaviors *preclude opportunities* for *negotiation* of mutually acceptable roles. Preclusion of opportunities for negotiating for mutually acceptable roles occurs especially when health providers "know" the stages and the patient and family do not.

Being confronted with the knowledge that death is inevitable creates a problem or crisis for all. Patients are faced with a new experience, that of dying, with no prior experience to rely on for assistance. Whether young or old, there is a major threat to life goals. Unresolved problems from the past, such as dependency, passivity, and identity, may be evoked, increasing the person's anxiety.

Other interactors also face a crisis since they are directly confronted with the dying of another. Like the dying person, they may have little or no prior experience with dying or death. In addition, they may not understand or accept that feelings of anger, frustration, guilt, and despair, as well as feelings of compassion, pleasure, hope, and love are evoked when caring for persons who are dying, just as they are when caring for those who are not dying.

Dying, or interacting with dying persons, evokes intense personal feelings. Although all interactors may experience intense feelings, there is no assurance that they are the *same* feelings, or that they will result in the same actions. *To cope effectively does not mean that all persons do or should cope in the same manner.*

Although there is no recipe for dying or for caring for the dying, there is a growing accumulation of knowledge about how people die and how interactors act and react to the label of dying and to those who are dying. The identification of a body of knowledge which identifies universal concerns and common problems related to the process of dying can offer guidelines for preparing for and living with dying, and for caring for dying people. This body of knowledge can be transmitted through socialization of both lay persons and health care providers.

DETACHED CONCERN

The importance of the role of confidant both to the dying person and to other interactors suggests the need for socialization of health care providers, especially nurses, in techniques for developing *detached concern* (15). Nurses who develop detached concern will be able to maintain objectivity while personalizing their approach. Essential aspects of detached concern include demonstrating understanding of the dying person and showing concern without denying the reality of the situation.

Detached concern is better understood by looking at two extremes of behavior: *complete detachment* and *overinvolvement*. In complete detachment, emotional distance is gained through professionalizing or intellectualizing the situation. Dying is made an impersonal, external problem, an object to be studied or treated. There is an appropriate plan for treatment and there is an appropriate way to die.

Overinvolvement in the life of the dying person or overidentification with the dying person is the opposite extreme of complete detachment. In many instances overinvolved health care providers use the situation to work through their own feelings, to rework prior death experiences, and to restore or increase their own self-esteem.

Lack of training for detached concern leads to expressions of anger and scape-goating behavior among health professionals, and to increased anxiety and stress for all interactors. For example, one overinvolved nurse spent an entire morning in tears, which was not only disconcerting to other interactors, but divided their focus between responding to the needs of the grieving nurse and accomplishing the expected functions related to caring for the dying patient and his family.

Another manifestation of the need for socialization for detached concern was the need to take days off from work. Nurses refer to "taking mental health days" which are sick days taken for the sole purpose of regaining their perspective before resuming their roles in caring for dying persons.

Physicians, like nurses, would benefit from deliberate socialization to caring for dying patients. Intraprofessional seminars which focus on understanding the social processes influencing the behaviors of dying patients and health care providers would be helpful to health care professionals. Understanding these processes should assist health care professionals in more effectively creating an interactional environment which allows all interactors to negotiate for more acceptable roles. It may, in addition, decrease the discord between physicians and nurses and contribute to the formation of mutual support systems.

At present, most seminars about dying and death are presented from a psychological perspective. The emphasis is on helping health care providers feel more comfortable talking about dying and death and communicating with dying patients. Thus, their primary goal is to decrease the taboo nature of the subject. Although important, focus on intrapsychic phenomena, to the exclusion of understanding social processes and environmental and situational factors, offers little in opportunities for learning effective behavioral or interactional alternatives necessary in caring for dying patients.

IMPLICATIONS FOR RESEARCH

Many more studies are needed to develop a body of knowledge upon which to base decisions regarding dying, death, and the care of dying people. The circumstances and processes surrounding dying people as well as the characteristics of the involved people, are equally important. For instance, what are the situational and individual characteristics which contribute to the selection of a confidant? Should the characteristics of the interactors be considered in patient care assignments? Could the patterns of living-dying be identified in other environments? Would other patterns or combinations of patterns be identified in different populations such as the aged or if data covered a longer time span? Are there relationships between the patterns of living-dying and other variables such as age, sex, ethnicity, and environment of care? Are stereotyped images of dying learned in early childhood and reaffirmed in ordinary social interaction? Do these stereotypes persist even when faced with dying? What are the hopes of dying people? Are they related to the patterns of living-dying? Can they be fostered? What are the benefits of dying to the dying people, to their families and friends, and to health care providers? There is so much more to investigate and to know about living-dying and death.

POSTSCRIPT

Conducting a study in the area of dying was fraught with emotional overtones. The nurse/researcher, no less than other people, was socialized to dying and death as taboo subjects. There was the initial uncertainty created by the feeling that it was presumptuous to intrude on the privacy of these dying persons. It soon became evident that it was ludicrous to perceive dying persons as different from others. They expressed the same hopes, aspirations, and fears as non-dying individuals.

The rewards of sharing these patients' last days far exceeded the costs in feelings of loss when they died. There is no intent to imply that the nurse/researcher was insulated from the sadness which surrounded the situations.

There is no question that the perceptions and feelings of the nurse/researcher are as important as the reactions of those who are dying in exploring the subject. It is suggested that the perceptions and feelings of the readers may color their interpretations even as they read this book.

It is not easy to entertain the thought of dying, to tell other people that death is near, or to respond to the announcement of another's dying. Fear and uneasiness are to be expected.

It is difficult to say good-bye.

REFERENCES

1. Alsop S: Stay of Execution, New York, J. B. Lippincott Company, 1973
2. Commission on Chronic Illness, Proceedings of the Conference on Preventive Aspects of Chronic Disease, Baltimore, March 12 – 14, 1951
3. Erickson K: Note on the Sociology of Deviance, Social Problems 9:308, 1962
4. Berger PL, Luckman T: The Social Construction of Reality, Garden City, New Jersey, Anchor Books/Doubleday, 1967
5. Smelser N: Theory of Collective Behavior, New York, The Free Press, 1962, pp. 270 – 312
6. Smelser: Collective Behavior, p. 270
7. Smelser: Collective Behavior, p. 271
8. McCall GJ, Simmons JL: Identities and Interactions: an Examination of Human Associations in Everyday Life, New York, The Free Press, 1966
9. Goffman I: Encounters: Two Studies in the Sociology of Interactions, Indianapolis, Bobbs-Merrill Company, 1961, pp. 7 – 81
10. Simmel G: The stranger. In Wolff KH (ed): The Sociology of Georg Simmel, New York, The Free Press, 1950, pp. 402 – 408
11. Simmel: The Stranger, p. 145
12. Glaser B, Strauss A: Temporal Aspects of Dying as a Nonscheduled Status Passage, Chicago, Aldine Publishing Company, 1970
13. Glaser, Strauss: Nonscheduled Status Passage
14. Kubler-Ross E: On Death and Dying, New York, The Macmillan Company, 1969
15. Martocchio BC: Death and dying in intensive care units. In Daly BJ (ed): Intensive Care Nursing—Current Clinical Nursing Series, Flushing, New York, Medical Examination Publishing Company, Inc., 1980, pp. 441 – 463

APPENDIX

Nursing Care Plans

The appendix includes examples of five nursing care plans, which are actual care plans. Biographical and other information has been changed to protect the identity of the subjects, while keeping the meaning intact.

Samples 1 and 2 are written on the same patient on two separate admissions to demonstrate the change in approach to one patient over time.

SAMPLE I

PATIENT INFORMATION/ASSESSMENT/NURSING CARE		Name	
House Officer:	**Admitting Nurse:**	Hospital #	Date Adm.
Diagnosis: Metastatic Squamous Cell Ca	**Procedure:** Date:	Service	Doctor
	Marital Status: S (M) W D Sep		Age
	Religion: C Baptized:	**In case of emergency notify:** Name: Relation:	
Does Patient Know? Yes **Condition:** Fair	**Last rites:** 10/25	Address: Phone:	

LIVING PATTERNS

Family members or significant others:
Husband c̄ children

Dwelling:

Occupation:
Former lab tech.

Prosthetic Aids:
Soft neck collar

Eating Patterns:
Appetite poor

Sleeping Patterns:
Sleeps in short naps, watches T.V. until the stations sign off

Bowel and Bladder Patterns
Output low
No bowel problems at present

SHORT TERM MEDICAL AND NURSING ORDERS

T
P, R } tid
B P

Other:
Notify HO — urine output ↓ 200 cc/hr

Weight: qod

Intake: √

Output: √

Diet and Fluids:
10/4 house
10/25 250 cc fluid q1h until MN
3 hrs jce of choice alternate
c̄ 1 hr H$_2$O (no tomato jce)

Allergies: None Known

Special Orders: Patient wishes:
Crush Tylenol + Bufferin — dissolve
in apricot jce — use straw
give Valium whole c̄ crackers

Activity and Positioning:
10/4 Up ad lib
10/15 Assistance needed

	Progress	Date

Nursing Assessment: Pleasant, frail, 48 yr. old woman c̄ large cancerous lesion on scalp, with alopecia, in constant pain. Aware of diagnosis and very poor prognosis, derives much support from husband (ō children) and belief in God. Knowledgable about disease, has had contact c̄ other dying patients through her work in hematology. Major fear concerns inability to be good wife.

Long Term Nursing Care Goals:
  Control of pain
  Support current physical adjustment and emotional
    acceptance
  Involve husband in care
  Prepare for future adjustments imposed by compli-
    cations

Teaching Plans:
  At this time pt. will not allow herself to make re-
    quests
  Reinforce idea that requests for care are:
  helpful
  expected
  necessary

Discharge Plans:
  Functional adaptation to home situation (re: appli-
    ances, hospital bed, housekeeping, etc.)
  Help in home—VNA referral and homemaker to do
    housework

Plans made c̄ social service for sitter to be c̄ patient 5 days/wk. Homemaker on Sat. Bed obtained

Date:	Patient Care Problems	Nursing Actions
	EMOTIONAL	
	1. Anxiety over medications, especially	Please reassure pt. @ 6 AM by telling her that you are giving her Dantroline & make a point of letting her know
	2. Emotional liability	A. Wishes to talk about illness—prefers use of word "cancer" B Stay with her if she appears depressed—prefers nonverbal reassurance, e.g., sit at bedside
	3. Need for independence, will not request help	A. Check position frequently—change throughout night (constant problem) will not request help B. Encourage alternative positions to make sure she is comfortable
	PHYSICAL	
	4. Conservation of strength	Enlist her participation in pacing activities; plan for rest periods; encourage visitors to space visits
	5. Weakness in shoulders and arms	A. Position tables so all articles are low (won't have to try to lift arm) B. Assist in combing hair C. Figure-8 sling to support arm
	6. Comfort	Pt. likes to take tub bath and use Alpha Keri lotion
	7. Safety	Make sure patient has help and does not slip trying to get out of tub by herself

APPENDIX

SAMPLE II

PATIENT INFORMATION/ASSESSMENT/NURSING CARE		Name	
House Officer:	Admitting Nurse:	Hospital #	Date Adm.
Diagnosis: 　Metastatic Squamous 　Cell Ca	Procedure:　Date:	Service	Doctor
	Marital Status: S (M) W D Sep		Age
	Religion:　C　Baptized:	In case of emergency notify: Name:　　　　Relation:	
Does Patient Know?　Yes Condition:　Poor	Last rites:	Address:　　　Phone:	

LIVING PATTERNS　　No Code Three

Family members or significant others:
　Husband c̄ children

Dwelling:

Occupation:
　Former lab tech.

Prosthetic Aids:

Eating Patterns:
　Sips of fluid, crackers

Sleeping Patterns:
　Naps only

Bowel and Bladder Patterns:
　Incontinent

SHORT TERM MEDICAL AND NURSING ORDERS

T ⎫
P, R ⎬ q shift
B P ⎭　　　Other:

Weight:

Intake:

Output:

Allergies:　None known

Special Orders:
　Crush Tylenol + Bufferin − dissolve
　in apricot jce, use straw
　Valium (don't crush) c̄ crackers

Diet and Fluids:
　Ad lib

Activity and Positioning:
　Ad lib c̄ help

157

	Progress	Date

Nursing Assessment:
  48 yr. old female readmitted for change in chemotherapy for Ca—past treatments ineffective. In constant pain, unable to care for self, sometimes disori-
  ented. Husband concerned over mental status,
  seems unaccepting of prognosis. Patient always attended by husband, mother-in-law, or sitter.

Long Term Nursing Care Goals:
  Provide for dignity and privacy
  Support family

Teaching Plans:

Discharge Plans:

Date:	Patient Care Problems	Nursing Actions
12/30	Skin care	A. Pt. is frequently incontinent—Keep dry; try to get M.D.'s order for catheter B. Use back-rub lotion C. Turn every 2 hours
	Comfort	A. Use pillow to support spine B. Keep medicated every 4 hours C. Likes frequent sips of cold ginger ale D. Alternate IM injection sites
	Support of husband and family	A. Try not to medicate patient right before visits, so patient will be more alert B. Help husband understand need for continued pain medication C. Encourage visitors to stay and help explain patient's behavior as necessary D. Help family with concern over husband's reactions
	Emotional support	A. Keep rosary near patient B. Pray with patient when she requests C. When patient is alert—give her chance to make her own decisions about care

SAMPLE III

PATIENT INFORMATION/ASSESSMENT/NURSING CARE		Name	
House Officer:	Admitting Nurse:	Hospital #	Date Adm.

Diagnosis:
   Pelvic Fx
   Anemia
   Multiple myeloma
	Procedure: Date:	Service	Doctor

	Marital Status: S M (W) D Sep		Age
	Religion: P Baptized:	In case of emergency notify: Name: Relation:	
Does Patient Know? No Condition:	Last rites:	Address: Phone:	

LIVING PATTERNS

Family members or significant others:
   Widowed, has 3 grown children in
   Cleveland

Dwelling:
   Lives alone in her home

Occupation:
   Housekeeper, has not worked since
   6/74

Prosthetic Aids:
   Walker

Eating Patterns:
   Does own cooking or has family
   bring food to her when she is not
   feeling well.

Sleeping Patterns:
   No difficulty in sleeping in the hospital. Sometimes difficulty sleeping
   at home because of leg pain.

Bowel and Bladder Patterns
   ō diff c̄ urination BM qd takes
   MOM for occasional constipation

SHORT TERM MEDICAL AND NURSING ORDERS

T ⎫
  ⎪ tid
P, R ⎬   Posturals
  ⎪ qid
B P ⎭

            Other:

Weight:

Intake: √

Output: √

Diet and Fluids:
9/20
   2 gm Na diet

Allergies:

Special Orders:
   9/22 weigh today
   9/30 discharge in AM

Activity and Positioning:
   9/20 OOB → chair if possible
          bedside commode
   No wt. bearing (L) foot

	Progress	Date

Nursing Assessment:
   59 yr old widow who fell off footstool in June,
74 while @ work—Dx pelvic fx. She was not able to
continue work p̄ fall because of pain. 1 wk PTA
pain ↑ & became worse—she became weak & unable to get OOB. Ambulates c̄ walker but needs asst.
getting OOB.
   She is alert & friendly. She receives much support from family & relatives. She does not know
about Dx of multiple myeloma.

Long Term Nursing Care Goals:
   9/25 Will be discharged on 2 gm Na NAS diet. Dieti-
tian has spoken c̄ pt. & her daughters, she had diet
instructions.

Teaching Plans:

Discharge Plans:
   9/25 Plans to return to her own home p̄ discharge.
Will move bed from upstairs down to living room.
Will return to clinic 3x each wk for X-ray therapy.

Date:	Patient Care Problems	Nursing Actions
9/25	Safety—increased chance of injury due to weakness from anemia; demineralization of bones, increasing chance of fracture	1. Assist in & out of tub 2. Walker for ambulation—Keep walker near bed (it is her *Own* walker) 3. No Ⓛ foot weight bearing
	Possible impaired renal function—due to cast cells in kidney	Careful I & O—pt. is on Lasix and Alkeran Note any decrease in output—Alkeran is excreted per kidney and cumulative effects can occur with decreased output Force fluids (likes Sanka, fr. jce)
	Increased chance of infection due to abnormal antibody production	Keep all personnel and visitors with URI's away from patient Teach patient to avoid exposure to others with URI's Teach pt. to obtain immediate care for cuts, abrasions, etc.

SAMPLE IV

PATIENT INFORMATION/ASSESSMENT/NURSING CARE			Name	
House Officer:	Admitting Nurse:		Hospital #	Date Adm.
Diagnosis: 9/27 SP MI	Procedure: Date:		Service	Doctor
	Marital Status: S M (W) D Sep			Age
	Religion: J Baptized:		In case of emergency notify: Name: Relation:	
Does Patient Know? Yes Condition: 9/27 Fair	Last rites:		Address: Phone:	

LIVING PATTERNS

Family members or significant others:
    1 daughter in Cleveland, 1 in Flor-
    ida; lives with companion, middle
    aged, for past yr.
Dwelling: she does housekeeping
            cooking & "looks after" pt.
            They live in an apartment.

Occupation:
    Formerly housewife

Prosthetic Aids:
    Glasses for reading

Eating Patterns:
    3 meals/day
    frozen food, often

Sleeping Patterns:
    c̄ difficulty—naps during day

Bowel and Bladder Patterns
    BM qd

SHORT TERM MEDICAL AND NURSING ORDERS

T   9/30 qid   Other:

P, R

B P

Weight: qd

Intake:

Output:

Allergies:

Special Orders:
    9/27 Telemetry

Diet and Fluids:
    9/27 1500 cc   750/750
    9/27 NAS house
    9/29 2000 cc   1000/1000

Activity and Positioning:
    10/3 up in chair 2 hr tid
    10/4 walk in hall c̄ asst.

	Progress	Date

Nursing Assessment:
Alert 87 yr. old adm. to hospital for chest pain dx as MI. Had been home—1 day $\bar{p}$ previous adm. for cardiac insuff. Widowed for 2 years, lives with companion in apartment.

Long Term Nursing Care Goals:

Teaching Plans:

Discharge Plans:
Pt. plans to return to aprt. $\bar{c}$ companion. Companion conscientious & interested in pt. (visits qd) Daughters keep in close contact $\bar{c}$ pt.

Date:	Patient Care Problems	Nursing Actions
	ADL, Rest Extremely weak and tires easily	Up in chair tid for 2 hrs—likes meds when sitting up. 2 people needed to transfer pt. to chair—she does not bear much wt.
	Depressed re: dependence needs since MI	Allow choices in care Rx times, when she wants to get up Point out her abilities to do things, e.g., wash face—point out progress as it appears
	Frightened about health → overly cooperative and solicitous with staff "I'll do anything you say"	↑ her security by letting patient know which staff she will be seeing, when they will return Keep bell cord in reach Give choices on care

SAMPLE V

PATIENT INFORMATION/ASSESSMENT/NURSING CARE	Name

House Officer:	Admitting Nurse:	Hospital # Date Adm.

Diagnosis:
  11/19:
  Renal failure dialysis
  seizures

Procedure: Date:	Service Doctor

| Marital Status: S (M) W D Sep | Age |

Religion: J   Baptized:

11/19
Does Patient Know? Yes   Last rites:
Condition: Guarded

In case of emergency notify:
Name: Relation:

Address: Phone:

LIVING PATTERNS

Family members or significant others:
  Father

Eating Patterns:
  Appetite good

Dwelling:

Sleeping Patterns:
  See note

Occupation:
  Dentist

Bowel and Bladder Patterns

Prosthetic Aids: Leave night light on to prevent visual hallucinations. No need for seizure precautions

SHORT TERM MEDICAL AND NURSING ORDERS

T
P, R } qs
B P

Other:

Diet and Fluids:
  2000 mg Na
  60 mg K
  60 mg Pro

  11/20 No fluid restriction

Weight: wt. qod

Intake:
Output: } 11/19

Allergies: None Known

Special Orders:
  11/19 Stool & Needle Precautions
  Call HO 90/50 < BP > $\frac{180}{105}$ 55 < P > 120
Private Rm when available

Activity and Positioning:
  Ad lib—encourage activity—needs assistance getting out of bed and walking

	Progress	Date

Nursing Assessment:

35 yr old dentist who has had chronic renal disease since early 20's and has progressed to needing hemodialysis for life maintenance. He is able to regulate his own diet & fluids. About July of this yr. he noted tremors on face & occas. forgetful spells. During the intervening months he has developed focal seizures of the face esp. about the tongue & mandible/maxilla. Pt seems able to handle secretions. Is oriented during seizure activity, though more recently relates difficulty remembering recent wants/names, feels lethargic & sleepy & feels ataxic. Gait stability of concern.

Long Term Nursing Care Goals:

Lives c̄ wife & 2 sons (9,7 yrs). Relates he is very frightened of permanency of this disability; states at times he feels he is losing his grip on his mentation. Also the patient is fearful about his job. States he is a dentist and while he is gone his assistant does the job but he just can't carry on as if he were there.

Teaching Plans:

Discharge Plans:

Date:	Patient Care Problems	Nursing Actions
11/21	1. Fluid balance—output 250 – 350 cc	1. Does better managing own fluid balance *Should gain 1 kg between ∼ dialysis let pt regulate fluids to est. this 1 kg gain—24° intake should be 1000 – 1200 cc recheck c̄ pt—some memory loss for recent events Diet NAS home & pt will select proper food
11/21	2. Seizure control & protection of pt; seizures worse p̄ dialysis	2. Light cord within reach all times Observe duration, extent of involvement behavior during seizures IV Valium per physician has been only control of seizures so far Pt can communicate well in writing during seizures
11/21	3. Pt awareness of health problem	3. Very aware of mental decline & is frightened voicing fear of permanence of symptoms—Handle by listening & reflecting actions/ treatments approaches back to his discussions with his physicians. At particularly stressful times may try to reach Dr. _____, psychiatrist who is seeing him Allow pt to verbalize his fears for his practice, future dialysis, etc.
11/21	4. Adequacy of rest	4. Has much diff resting in hosp. due to care interruptions rather than inability to sleep for most part Group Rx together & maintain flexibility in Rx & med sched.

Date:	Patient Care Problems	Nursing Actions

Dialysis Schedule

1. *Meds*
   a. Hold *multivits* & *Folate* til p̄ treatment (these are dialyzed out)
   b. Hold *Aldomet* AM dose prior to dialysis
   c. Alucaps, Colase will be given in dialysis unit
   d. PRN's will be charted on med sheet—please send c̄ pt

2. *Meals*
   a. Make arrangements day prior to have *breakfast* & *lunch* trays sent to dialysis unit.

3. *I&O*
   a. I&O will be kept & recorded on pts fluid balance sheet for the day— please send c̄ pt.

4. *Blood & Other Specs*
   a. Send requisitions for any AM bloods needed to dialysis unit & will be drawn there. Please identify by note on chart or call attn to these.

*5. *Dialysis times*
   T, Th, Sat 8 AM → 1 PM Please have on unit @ 8 AM. We will call you to tell you when he's ready to return to the floor.

6. *PreCare*
   Do daily wt on floor
   Call & give oral report to dialysis unit—any special care problem needs.

7. *PostCare*
   Will call report back to you. Bandages on fistula came off following AM. No heat to fistula for 12 hours p̄ dialysis. Resume floor care routine. Pt may experience nausea, headaches, seizures p̄ rx → support c̄ comfort measures & prn meds. Nausea & headaches may take several hours to clear and are due to the changes in fluid & solute balance in extra- & intracellular fluids.

INDEX

contrary action to, penalties and rewards
from, 104
sign of, 83
Unnatural death, research on, 29 — 30
Unwitnessed death, 23

Value(s), 21
  internalization of, 42
  related to dying and death, 1
Value system, 139
Victory, over death, 10
Vie et Mort (Bichat), 14
Violent death, 22
Virtue, rewards from, 8
Visiting, patterns of, 64 — 65
Visiting hour(s)
  dying patient label and, 98, 99
  hospital policy on, 63
Visitor(s), 41, 52, 60, 99, 115, 118
  family and significant others

hospital policy and practice on, 63 — 64
patients' feelings on, 63, 64
patterns of visits, 64 — 65
socialization of, 105
Vovelle, M., 15

Wahl, C.W., 22
Weisman, A.D., 32
Well aged, 68
Western society, 3
Will(s)
  changes in, 15
  living, 27
  roles of, 15
  see also Last Will and Testament
Withdrawal behavior, *see* Avoidance behavior
Working agreement(s), 117
  purpose of, 144
  reaching of, 144
  role negotiation through, 129